Introducing

YOGA

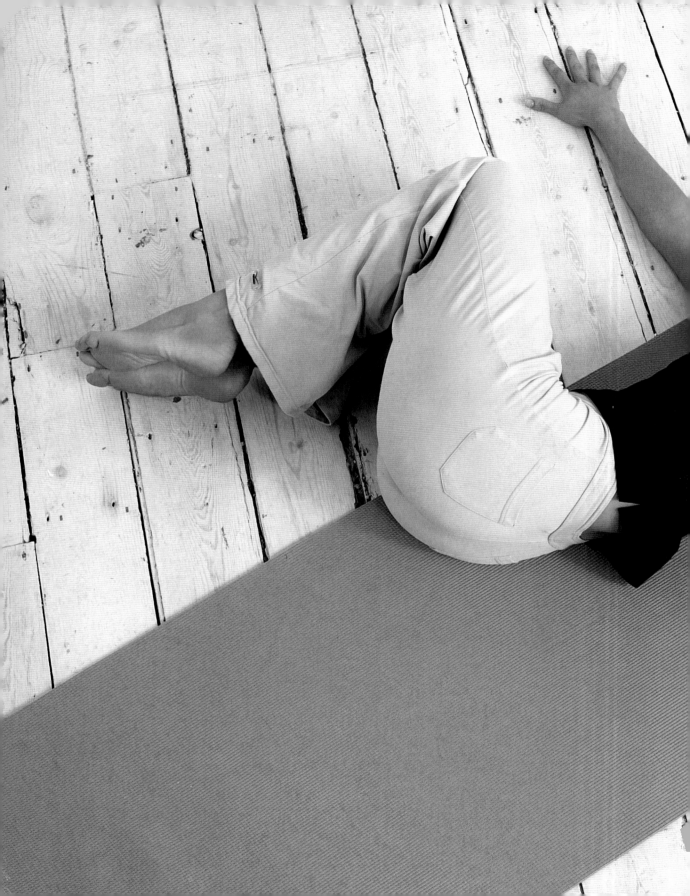

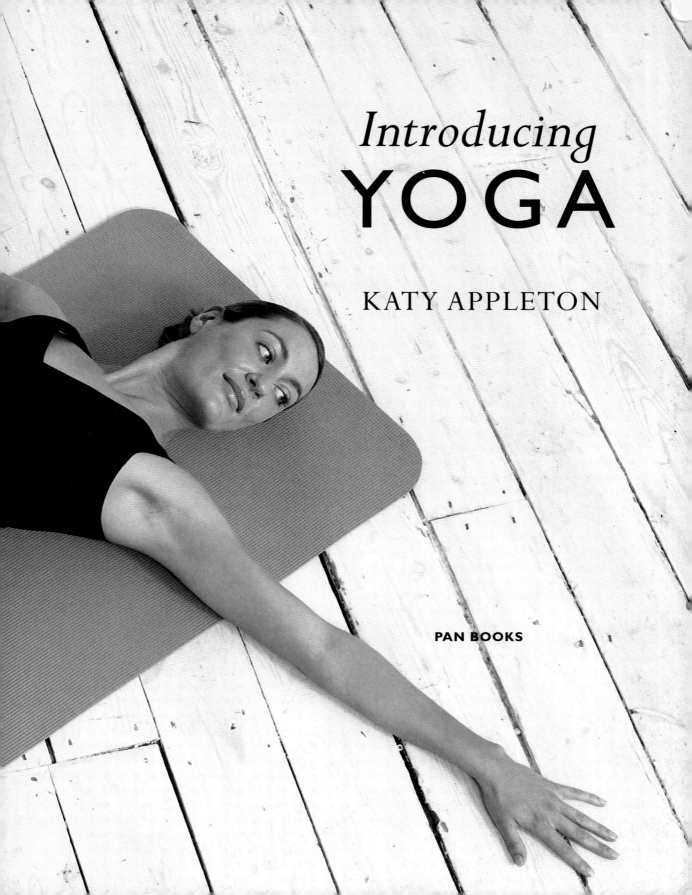

Introducing
YOGA

KATY APPLETON

PAN BOOKS

First published 2002 by Pan Books
an imprint of Pan Macmillan Publishers Ltd
Pan Macmillan, 20 New Wharf Road, London N1 9RR
Basingstoke and Oxford
Associated companies throughout the world
www.panmacmillan.com

ISBN 0 330 41204 3

1 3 5 7 9 8 6 4 2

A CIP catalogue record for this book is available from the British Library.

Designed by Peter Ward
Photography by Jim Marks
Illustrations © Becky Halls, 2002
Printed and bound by Butler and Tanner of Frome and London

CONTENTS

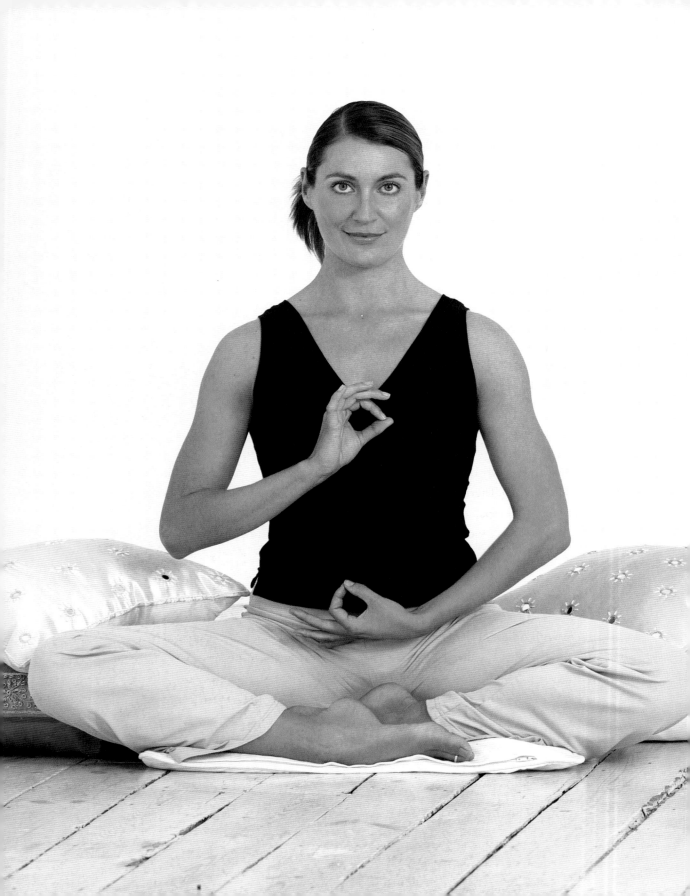

INTRODUCTION

Welcome to *Introducing Yoga*. To start with, I would like to explain how I took my first steps towards yoga and how you can use this book to begin your own journey.

My mother did yoga when she was pregnant with me, which must be how I caught the yoga bug. However, my early childhood experiences of yoga only consisted of being taken to a few classes with my mum. When I was quite young, at the age of eleven, I left home to go to ballet school to train as a classical dancer, and at seventeen I became a professional dancer. Within a year I knew I needed something to balance the very physical demands of dance. Ballet is incredibly beautiful and magical, but I found the environment sometimes frustrating. There is a huge emphasis on how you should look, and directors of ballet companies expect you to eat, sleep and breathe dancing. Although I adored my dancing career, I found I was beginning to lose touch with who I was. I began to take time out to be by myself and sit quietly and breathe. Little did I know at the time that this is the essence of yoga. The quiet breathing and relaxation brought an incredible peace and balance into my very hectic life. These tools of yoga were a great gift, and I felt I wanted to share them with others. I decided to do a yoga teacher training course and when I'd finished this I realized that practising yoga was going to become a way of life for me. The more my own life became centred around yoga and the more I taught others, the more it became obvious to me that the benefits of yoga can be felt by anyone, irrespective of age, sex, shape or lifestyle. All

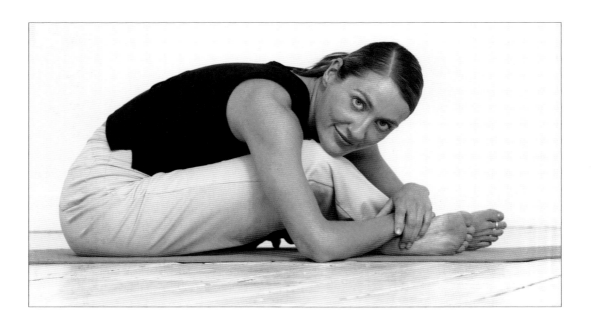

that is needed to begin with is a little discipline to make time each day for your own practice, even if it's only for a few minutes, and to become aware of the movements of the body and breath. After a while, the discipline becomes easy and you will find yourself creating time to practise and looking forward to it and the benefits it brings you.

It is always such a pleasure to see my students take their first steps in yoga and to share their enjoyment and wonder that something so simple can eliminate problems that may have been present for years, whether mental, physical or emotional. I have seen in myself and in others time and time again that yoga works on many different levels, and that the results are unique to each individual. I believe more than anything that this knowledge should be shared with everyone. That is why I decided to write this book to help guide you on your way. What you find on your journey will be personal to you.

Enjoy.

You can contact Katy through her website www.appleyoga.com

How to Use This Book

There are so many different yoga books available these days which show in great detail the many different postures available to the intermediate and advanced yoga student. But many of my students have said that initially they have been put off by yoga books, simply because they look too complicated. The more advanced yoga postures aren't something you can just do immediately, first you have to condition the body and mind in order to learn the basic postures and then work in a certain way. That is where this book comes in; it is meant to serve as a beginner's guide to help you towards learning more advanced levels of yoga should you wish to, or it will just give you a few ideas on how to bring stretching and breathing exercises into your life.

Your body is like a machine. It is a highly complex web of bones, muscles, nerves, organs and skin working through the mind, which is your body's control centre. Like any other machine it needs to be kept in tip-top condition and fed the correct fuel on an ongoing basis. When any part of the body experiences difficulties the efficiency of the entire machine is at risk. Your body, which is so unique and so sensitive to change, needs a well-stocked yoga tool box to take care of it. This book will help to explain how to open this tool box and how best the tools can be used. It will help combat all the aches and pains your body and mind endures every day. The postures of yoga are designed to stretch and lubricate the joints, muscles, ligaments, bones and tendons of your body by increasing circulation and flexibility. Such a tool box should contain the necessary tools for heating, cooling, recharging and toning the system, as well as keeping the control centre, the mind, clear and sharp. Yoga can serve as a complete tool box to strengthen areas of weakness and to keep your body at any desired level of performance: it tones and stretches the external body, massages all the internal organs and stills the mind to help you cope with the pressures of daily life.

I am continually dipping into my own yoga tool box. How I use the tools available depends on my circumstances and my mood. Each morning I use yoga to wake me by doing the Sun Salutation, which will be explained later in the book. During the day I may also use breathing techniques to ground and centre myself if I feel excited or irritated. It is interesting to observe how you breathe and to be aware of what the breath is doing. For example, can you remember the last time you were excited or nervous? Didn't you feel your heartbeat race and your breath quicken? This is because your mind and body are connected.

This book does not contain the entire yoga tool box. It wasn't intended to. It is the equivalent of a beginner's course in yoga, introducing you to the basic movements and ways of thinking without bombarding you with too much information or too many postures that would make a beginner struggle.

If you have a look through the book you will see that I have given you three sequences of postures to work with, starting with a lying sequence, then a seated sequence and finally a standing sequence. Then there is an introduction to the wonderful Sun Salutation exercise.

I would recommend that you start at the beginning of the book and slowly work your way through it, so you become familiar with each posture and how it feels. Remember that some of the postures will be a gift to your body and you may find them physically easy, while others may take longer to master and you will need to persevere. Once you are comfortable with the

4

lying, seated and standing sequences of poses, have a look at the Programmes for Life where the Daily Mini Plans will tell you how to make these postures flow from one to another, coordinating the movements with the breath. I have deliberately put them into small sequences for people who may have limited time, so if you only have ten minutes in your day you can pick one sequence to work on and know that you have still dedicated some time to yourself and to your yoga. You'll also find a small shiatsu section there to help with some of life's stresses.

The Sun Salutation is a challenge, so do make sure that you feel comfortable with the other postures in the book first; I have given you some tips on how to practise each posture which will definitely help. It is an amazing sequence, one that I do every day of my life and will continue to do so. If I'm short of time, I do one of the set groups of postures to warm up and then some rounds of Sun Salutation and that starts my day with a wonderful feeling that I can cope with anything that comes my way.

One of the most important things to remember when you practise is not to be afraid to experiment and perhaps mix up the sequences or maybe choose one posture that feels good for your body on that particular day and stay in it for perhaps ten minutes. There really are no set rules in yoga. Just enjoy what you are doing, give it your full attention, stay present in what you are working on, and keep focusing on the breath even if you can only take a few minutes for your practice.

Each individual is different. Yoga acknowledges this. The tool box is one that can be used at any time and in a variety of ways. As you become more comfortable in certain postures and more aware of your body, you will find there is no limit to the number of tools available to challenge you further. I have never met a yoga student, no matter how advanced, who said that yoga had stopped being a challenge. Indeed in time yoga often becomes more a mental than a physical challenge. To benefit you mentally, yoga provides you with a collection of tools such as mind training and breathing. These exercise the mind in the same way that the physical postures stretch and tone the body.

Yoga should be fun, twisting and stretching all your cares away. As your tool box of postures grows you will find your body and mind working in new and wonderful ways. Once this begins to happen you will feel so much better physically, and also have a much more positive attitude to life. Yoga requires as much practice and patience as any other physical or mental pursuit, but the rewards can be so much greater, as you will hopefully discover for yourself. This book is not one long programme, to be done in its entirety before any benefits can seen. Instead, it is a selection of building blocks that, if practised, can begin to stretch your body and mind giving you a firm foundation from which to move forward. You will not become a yoga master after reading this book and practising the postures described in it; for that you would need further guidance from an experienced teacher or the use of a more advanced book. Whether or not you wish to explore more advanced yoga, the tools provided here can help anyone fight the effects of ageing or illness or of lifestyles that require long hours of sitting or stress. Some of you may find the postures easy and it is for that reason that I have tried to incorporate some ideas on more advanced stretches.

Dip into the yoga tool box and see what you feel comfortable with. It is a pleasure and a thrill to explore the constant changes in your body and mind. You have the ability to use any of the tools required for any job you wish. Unlike your car, you cannot trade in your body for a newer model after a certain number of miles. Make sure your own tool box for life is full of the best possible equipment.

What is Yoga?

Most people die with their music
still locked up inside of them.
Benjamin Disraeli

For me yoga began with a few tentative steps. It has now become a way of life and something that fills me with constant happiness and wonder. I always feel as if I am sitting on a great secret that I want to share with everyone and I am sure that is how most yoga teachers feel. Each time I practise yoga I feel as if I am coming home after a long time away, refreshed, with a new set of eyes, a vibrant breath and a strong and relaxed body. Yoga has been, and continues to be, a source of inspiration in every part of my life.

The word yoga means to bring together, to combine or unite. The word comes from the ancient language Sanskrit, which originated in the north-western part of India. Sanskrit words are a fact of life when beginning to learn yoga. Many teachers use the Sanskrit names for postures but this can often be confusing if you are only at the beginning of your yoga journey. My own students have told me that they have been put off by the use of too many Sanskrit words. They are made to feel as if they were in a foreign country with no knowledge of the local dialect, and for that reason I am going to try to use layman's terms as much as possible. However, there are some Sanskrit words that are impossible to avoid, and it is much better for anyone interested in learning more about yoga to understand these words. Therefore, the Sanskrit

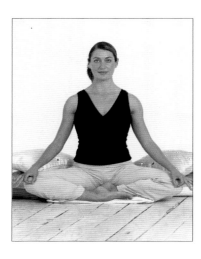

terms used in this book are ones I feel are important to the understanding of yoga, but they will be accompanied by a clear definition of the word and an explanation of how it fits into the whole picture.

Yoga unites your body and mind, the two aspects of your existence. It does this by working your body from within, gradually and calmly, in tune with your own natural harmony. How many times have you heard the expression 'a healthy person is a happy person'? By understanding the way your own body and mind works, you can begin to explore the connections inside yourself. Observing yourself, you can go from the physical, external body to the nerves, from the nerves to the senses, from the senses to the mind – it's an extraordinary journey. To understand the union between your body and mind is to begin to understand your own essence, spirit or soul. Through yoga you are able to embrace your soul and unlock the smile within.

The tree of yoga is made up of many, many different branches. Most students in the West come to yoga for the physical and mental benefits gained by practising the postures. The Sanskrit word for posture is asana. The practice of the physical postures or asanas is called Hatha Yoga which is the type of yoga discussed in this book, and is the style of yoga I have taught for almost five years. All you really need to know is that Hatha Yoga is a generic term for 'physical' yoga and is a combination of relaxation, breathing and postures. You may hear about all kinds of yoga taught at your local gym or done by celebrities, such as Iyengar, Bikrams, Ashtanga or Sivananda Yoga. It may seem confusing, but they are all part of Hatha Yoga – physical yoga. They all have different ideas on how the postures and breathing should be combined. In the final section of this book I will try and explain some of the basic differences between these types of yoga. As I mentioned before, all you

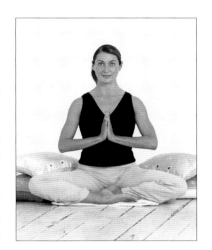

really need to know is that any yoga that works on your physical body is part of Hatha Yoga. Which style is right for you depends on what you want to achieve and how you want to get from A to Z on your yoga pathway. Choose which style is best for you, after all, nobody knows your body and mind like you do. Although I learned Sivananda-style yoga first, my teaching takes its influence from all the different styles taught in all the classes I have been to, and so I suppose I can be trendy and call this style of yoga, Hatha Fusion! I tend to combine different schools of yoga to suit what a particular student needs, and this is a theme I continually come back to when I'm teaching. Do what is right for you, and always be aware of what your body is telling you.

Yoga is a commitment to look after yourself better both mentally and physically. It is not asking you to change everything in your life or give up alcohol, or whatever it is you enjoy. Instead, it is about complementing the life you already lead, bringing an enhanced feeling of health, strength and peace to your daily routine. No matter what physical condition you are currently in, yoga can be a shining light to take you forward in life, so that you can develop naturally and deepen your relationship with everything around you. One of my first teachers taught disabled people for many years and found the enjoyment they got from yoga to be as great as that of any able-bodied person. Such moments will often be a teacher's greatest inspiration. It doesn't matter what you can and cannot do, only that you are committed to work towards improvement.

If you read more or talk to other people doing yoga, you may also hear about more branches of yoga such as Jnana Yoga or Raja Yoga. Don't worry; it is not as daunting as it may sound at first. Yoga is all about exploring the self, and exercising the physical body and mind is just one way of doing that.

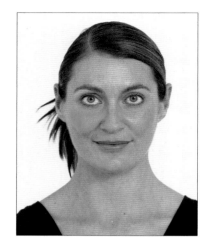

People who practise these other forms of yoga have simply found that they suit them better. There is no right way or wrong way. I know my own love of Hatha Yoga comes from my experiences as a ballet dancer, in fact I wish I had known more about the asanas when I was dancing professionally!! How amazed I would have been at the effects of yoga on the movement of the body and the breath. The movement of my body and breath always fascinated me, so Hatha Yoga was a natural path for me to take. You could say that yoga is just about finding a calmer place mentally, but I think that in our Western upbringing, which has a very physical culture, there tends to be a natural disposition towards the Hatha side of yoga in our societies. In India, a country where deep spirituality, contemplation and religion has existed amongst the people for thousands of years, Hatha Yoga is nowhere near as dominant as it is in Europe and North America.

Yoga is not about physical acrobatics. The point of Hatha Yoga is to find the limits of what you are able to do each time you make the commitment to practise. There is no competition in yoga, not even with yourself. If you are fighting against your body, then you will not be able to understand it. You simply do what you are able to do at that moment. In my own practice at the moment, headstands are not entirely comfortable for me to do. I could do a headstand if I had to, but why do things which your body is uncomfortable with? I know that in time my body will tend to itself and correct what is wrong, provided that I do not push it into a position it does not want to be in. Not being able to do specific postures does not make you any less of a yoga student. Flexibility is something that comes with patience and perseverance. Many friends of mine who have done yoga for a number of years still find it a constant source of amazement to observe that their bodies change internally and externally just as much, if not more, now than when they began their

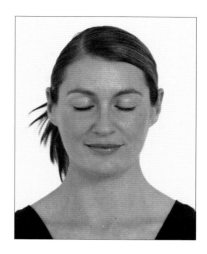

yoga journey. Just like life, you get out of yoga exactly what you put in. The great thing about yoga is that with each small step you take, the inspiration you get from, and the enjoyment of learning about your body grows in leaps and bounds. You will start to observe changes more and more quickly, and the inspiration and the enjoyment will begin to spill over into everything you do.

Do you have the time for yoga? Of course you do. Just slow down for a moment and think of how much time we spend every day thinking about nothing in particular, or in front of the television, or in bed before we get up in the morning. We all have time we could make for our health and well-being, and at first it can be a matter of minutes rather than hours. In time, you will find yourself creating space in your day for yoga, and you will wonder what you used to do with that time. Yoga is about seeing the distractions of the external world for what they are really worth, about learning to live in the current moment instead of dwelling in the past or dreaming about the future. One of my first teachers asked me, 'What do you want from life?' After a moment's thought I replied, 'Just to stay present.' Yoga has shown me how to live in the precious present. We all want to be present, in the moment and enjoying this life; this book can begin to open the doors to a wonderful way of living, feeling and experiencing. It won't take you all the way there by any stretch of the imagination, but hopefully it will introduce you to a new friend that can stay by your side for the rest of your life.

Find the harmony of your own body; you will thank yourself for it.

11

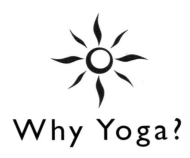

Why Yoga?

Moments of life are gift-wrapped in bright colours.

When you choose to practise yoga regularly your concentration and your memory will improve, and you will find more time for important things and less time for trivia. Your eating and digestion will get better and you will feel much more relaxed. Generally, your health and your whole outlook will improve, and with this will come a renewed excitement for life.

Why choose yoga when there are so many different activities to choose from? Yoga is just one way of exercising our physical bodies but many people are becoming aware that exercising only our physical body is not enough to attain total fitness. Our body and mind are like two parts of the same machine, and we need to find ways of ensuring that time is devoted to exercising both. Most traditional Western physical activity is of a sporting nature, involving competition and violent impacts that resonate in the body long after they have occurred. Holistic approaches to health and physical fitness, such as yoga, view the body and mind as one, and look to work on both at the same time and in equal ways. This can be done directly (through physical exercise) or indirectly (through mind control and awareness of breath). Yoga is the most complete approach to personal health and growth ever created by human beings. On its own or as a complement to other fitness regimes, yoga can unlock the full potential of your body and mind, creating new space for you to achieve anything you set your mind to.

The main differences between yoga and Western physical exercise should be understood. Yoga does not encourage violent muscle movement (such as repeated starting and stopping, sudden turns and physical contact) because such movement causes the muscles to become tired and stiff. Every part of our body requires a fresh intake of oxygen to replenish it. As we exercise, our muscles need more oxygen than our inhalation may be able to provide. The difference between the amounts of oxygen our muscles need and the amount our inhalation provides is called our 'oxygen debt'. Without proper relaxation and breathing to pay off the oxygen debt caused by physical exertion, something called lactic acid begins to accumulate in the muscles and blood, causing muscle tiredness to set in. When the body is tired and not properly stretched, then the likelihood of injuries increases dramatically. Our bodies can be likened to musical instruments – they need to be in tune in order to give the maximum performance possible. You see, yoga regards your physical body as an instrument with which to achieve higher states of consciousness. When our bodies and minds are in perfect tune together, it becomes easier to clarify our thoughts and achieve a higher state. Physical exercise in the West is viewed as helping the body withstand the daily toils of life, or as a fashion statement, or as a weapon to be launched at an opponent. The body and mind do not work in harmony, and therefore the mind is seldom in control.

The foundations of yoga are breathing, posture and relaxation.

BREATHING

Hatha Yoga works on the body both internally and externally, linking the body and mind through the breath, which is considered to be the essence of life itself. We all need air to live. Breathing gives life: it replenishes your system, and balances your emotions. Your cardiovascular and respiratory systems are the way that oxygen and nutrients enter the body tissues and vital organs through inhalation, and the removal of gaseous waste products of the body is through exhalation. Your bodies were designed for deep, abdominal, rhythmic breathing. Too many of us never experience the joy and benefits of proper full breathing, instead breathing shallowly. Yoga focuses on the breath and teaches us to be aware of it. Through understanding the breath, we understand the movement of the life force through our body and we bring calm into our minds and our lives.

POSTURES

When our breathing is deep and regulated, the body is working naturally in the most efficient way, and is able to move in tune with the breath. Yoga uses various combinations of asanas (postures) to stretch and strengthen the entire system. The asanas should be done slowly and comfortably, with awareness of your limits, both in terms of flexibility and of stamina. In time, you will find your limits expanding, and physical blockages disappearing. By understanding your physical nature better, you will also begin to see your mental nature more clearly.

RELAXATION

As mentioned before, physical exercise can cause muscle tiredness when your body requires more oxygen than it is getting. Yoga uses long periods of relaxation to counter the effects of oxygen debt. But the benefits of relaxation before, during and after asana practice are much greater than simply countering tiredness. Modern life is not geared towards relaxation. For many of us, relaxation is sitting in front of the television with a glass of wine in our hand. Now there is nothing wrong with that, but could you really call it relaxation? True relaxation is to let go of everything for a time, and simply to rest in the natural state of the breath, this state being unforced, relaxed and slowly rhythmic. Thoughts are just allowed to come and go and the body is allowed to sink into a relaxed, centred state. It is no surprise that the most basic posture in yoga relaxation is called the Corpse Pose, savasana in Sanskrit. Discipline of the mind is impossible without relaxation; how can our mind relax if our bodies are tense, irritated and active?

When practising yoga, patience and a proper approach will always lead to great physical and mental benefits. My advice would be: don't set any goals for your yoga practice, or if you do need to set a goal don't set it too high in case you are disappointed if you don't achieve it. Just observe what your body is capable of now, and watch it change from day to day, week to week and year to year. On some days your body may want to move more than on other days. On some days it just won't want to move at all, in which case you can always focus more on the breathing or mind-training techniques that are described in this book. Never be too excited and never get frustrated. Instead, observe the entire body and try to understand your changing nature. You know that when you are happy you tend to feel better both mentally and physically. Yoga allows you to understand this connection and, in time, to achieve greater balance and consistency both in your yoga practice, and in life itself.

We are all made up of energy. It just happens that your energy has come together as a human being this time around. Modern physics has proved we are creatures of energy in recent years but it has been acknowledged in the practice of yoga for thousands of years. The theory of yoga is that the energy within the body is exactly the same as the energy that makes up everything in the universe. The air you breathe is pure energy, or prana. Through breathing, posture and relaxation you are able to create space within your body for energy to flow freely.

The mental and physical blockages within your system stop the free flow of energy through your body. All your life you have been creating these blockages. Look upon them as part of your personality. For instance, a traumatic childhood experience would certainly manifest itself in some sort of mental block, however, so too would a happy childhood experience. The blockages are not good or bad; they simply exist and stop the free flow of energy. Physical blockages are more apparent. You can feel them as you move. But mental blockages are there as well, and sometimes they cause you far greater discomfort than the physical kind. Mental blockages occur when you allow your emotions or your ego to control you, leading to states of extreme happiness or despair, love or hatred, strength or weakness. All these extremes unbalance you and, in the same way that improper use of the body causes physical blockages, lead to mental blockages growing within your system, imprinted with the trials and tribulations of life, often manifesting themselves as further physical aches and pains.

Yoga gradually eliminates all the various blockages from the system, layer by wonderful layer. You can feel the body and mind opening out, blossoming and becoming free. Mental and physical baggage no longer needed is set loose and, as the blockages are cleared, then the prana, the energy of life, can flow freely through your system. You will feel this energy as well. There is nothing secret about it, and it doesn't take a lifetime of dedicated practice to achieve. At first you probably won't even realize it is happening. Unfortunately, explaining how it will feel is almost impossible, as the sensation is unique to each person. This is what is meant when yoga teachers talk about understanding the body and being aware of how it is changing.

A commitment, however great or small to yoga will create mental discipline. Actually practising yoga creates physical strength and a feeling of health and well-being. Once these are felt, you will want to continue and your practice will become free from effort. This feeling will just creep up on you, I promise!

Will yoga help you deal with problems such as stress or tiredness? Definitely yes, if you give it time and commitment. I have never met anyone who did yoga who didn't say that it had helped them every day of their life. You will begin to see the stress dissolve, your sleeping will improve, your eating become more enjoyable and your relationships deepen. Changes will be there in everything you do. And change is fact, isn't it? It is happening all the time around you.

I am often asked whether yoga helps in weight loss. Of course it can if done properly and regularly. But loss of weight and improvements in physical appearance are just side benefits, and not the main point of yoga. For instance, the thyroid gland, located in the neck, is an endocrine gland that directly balances the body's metabolic rate and metabolic rate influences your weight control and stamina. There are very few ways in Western physical culture to stimulate this gland, but there are several yoga asanas that directly stimulate it. Everything in yoga is about bringing you to your natural state, in harmony with yourself and everything around you.

Yoga will make you feel fantastic. You don't need a lot of space, you don't need to spend money joining a gym, and you certainly don't need to worry about what others will think of your physical condition. It is a tool that can travel anywhere with you, and you won't need to make any extra effort to carry it. Don't buy the book and allow this wonderful gift to sit gathering dust. As the saying goes, 'Just do it!'

Ten Stepping Stones
Towards Yoga Practice

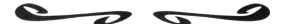

1. I would definitely suggest buying a proper yoga mat, as there is a real risk of slipping on any other surface. A proper mat is not expensive and does make a difference. Most people end up feeling very protective of their yoga mat! Wear comfortable clothes that your body can move in freely. Yoga is normally practised in bare feet.

2. Try to create the same space in your home to practise in every day. If you can keep your mat on the floor all the time do so, as this will remind you to step on it . . . but if you don't have the space to do that, put your mat somewhere clearly visible to gently prompt you to do your practice.

3. Turn off your telephones, make a mental note that no one can disturb you while you are practising. Don't have the TV on. A little music can sometimes be inspiring. I go through phases where I love to have music and at other times I turn the music on and all it does is distract me, so off it goes! Find what works for you.

4. Create a comfortable atmosphere for yourself. You might like to light a candle, or maybe some incense, or even an oil burner. Sometimes I do this when I have had a long day and need soothing! If it's space I need I often open a window and take away the clutter from the room. There are loads of things you can do to feel clearer, these are of course just a few suggestions.

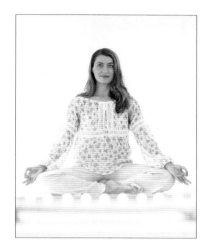

5.   Try and do ten minutes daily. Everybody has time for that. You may find you keep going just because it feels so great.

6.   You should leave two hours minimum after eating before you start to practise. And please, never attempt any yoga if you have been drinking alcohol.

7.   If you have any long-standing injuries or illnesses please consult your doctor before you begin any yoga.

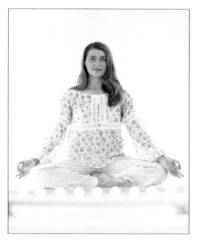

8.   This book isn't written with pregnant women in mind, although yoga during pregnancy is wonderful. If you have recently become pregnant and wish to start yoga, I would suggest finding a teacher who has experience in dealing with yoga and pregnancy.

9.   Be aware of how you are feeling when you start your practice. It will always be different. Sometimes the energy will be high, sometimes a little low, so listen to what your body is telling you. There is no competition in yoga, with yourself or others. Make a mental note that this time is for you and you alone.

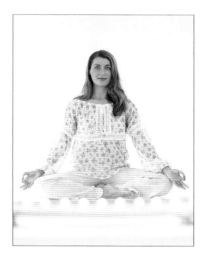

10. The mind loves to wander to the past or the future; try and stay in the present moment when you practise. I keep my mind on the breath, observing what it's doing and how it feels. By doing this my mind stays in the now.

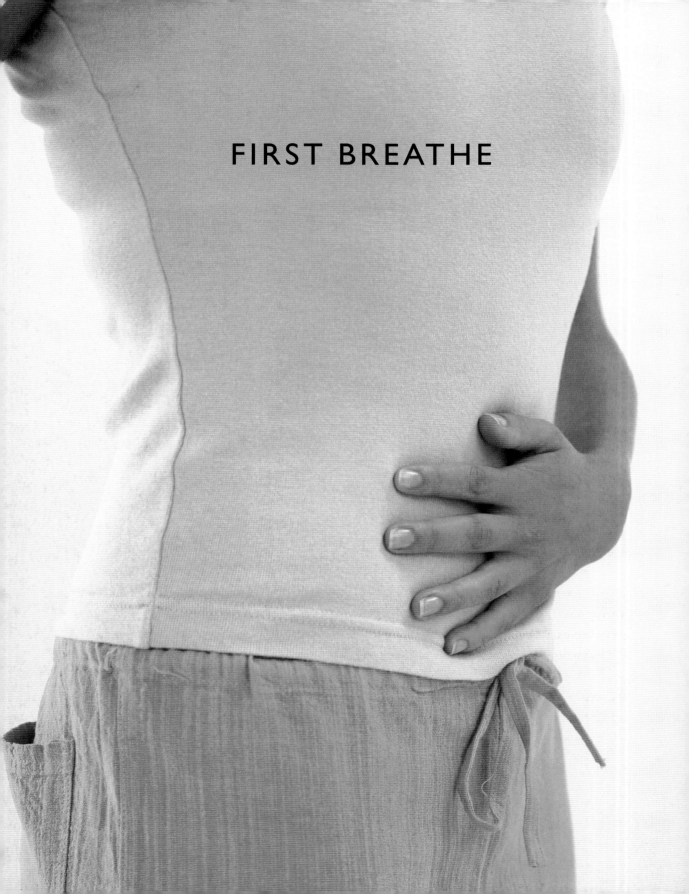

FIRST BREATHE

Breathing

We all breathe. Without breath there would be no human life. However, despite its obvious importance breathing is something many of us simply allow to happen unconsciously, as if there was no need to nurture or care for the breath. Because of this, our breathing habits become poor, and the majority of us use only a small portion of our full lung capacity in our normal inhalation and exhalation. We breathe shallowly, lifting only a little of the ribcage and with our shoulders hunched which allows only a fraction of the air available to filter down into and through our bodies.

In yoga the breath is equal to the energy of life. Breathing is not just a matter of allowing oxygen and other nutrients into our system, neither is it just a tool to expel waste gases from our system through exhalation. The breath is life itself. For me, breathing is like a dance, something beautiful and inspiring. Every time you breathe, you take in the essence of existence, the energy of the universe. Control of breathing concentrates the vital nerve energy, leading to increased control of the body and mind.

Even modern medicine acknowledges the importance of proper breathing to fight diseases of the body and mind. For centuries the flow of the breath, or prana, through the body has been central to all forms of holistic medicine such as acupuncture and shiatsu.

The link between the body and breath is obvious enough. Under severe physical exertion our pulse tends to quicken and we become short of breath. This is due to the fact our muscles need oxygen to perform any activity and when we exercise, our muscles require much more oxygen than our normal breathing provides. Unconsciously our body tells us to consume more oxygen and consciously we may react by quickening our breathing. In yoga we learn that this quickening of the breathing does not provide more oxygen to the muscles, as most of us simply inhale and exhale more quickly rather than actually taking in more oxygen. Proper breathing is about feeling the movement of the inhalation build up deep in the diaphragm, allowing the oxygen to flow throughout your body, then slowly and just as deeply exhaling, pushing the new energy throughout your body while at the same time expelling carbon dioxide from your lungs. By controlling your breathing in this manner you will find that you are receiving all the oxygen your muscles require, without having to quicken your breath or stop the activity you are performing.

There is also a link between the mind and our breath, although we may not be aware of it. When you concentrate deeply, your breathing tends to slow down and lengthen, sometimes it may stop entirely for a time. Likewise, when you are agitated or bothered, breathing speeds up and becomes shallow and disjointed. Our breath also affects the state of our mind. By slowing our breathing, and controlling the inhalation and exhalation consciously, we are able to clear the mind and listen to the pulse of our body, the pulse of the universe.

BREATHING TECHNIQUES

It sounds so easy doesn't it? We are constantly breathing and often entire days will pass without us even once thinking about how we are doing it. The techniques described here are by no means advanced, and may be practised by anyone. However, the benefits gained from taking time to be aware of how we breathe are enormous. Give yourself ten minutes or so to try these techniques and continue to practise them as often as possible. There may be days when your nose is blocked and breathing is difficult; please don't use that as an excuse not to practise. Over time you will discover that sinus problems are alleviated, breathing becomes deeper and more natural, and the entire body feels energized and healthy. Use the air you breathe to find a more comfortable place for your body and mind to rest.

Always practise breathing in a comfortable position. This can be flat on your back, seated or even standing. I will be teaching you three basic breathing techniques and will recommend a position in which to practise each one of them. But remember, listen to your own body and if you feel uncomfortable and unable to concentrate properly on your breathing, then try another position. The most important thing is that your spine should be as straight as possible and your chest should be opened. To accomplish this, pull your shoulders back slightly and feel your chest expand. Don't push the shoulders back too far; just let them fall back in line with the torso. Take a look at how many people walk around with their shoulders slouched forward. Think about what this is doing to their lungs and spine. It constricts their breathing and curves the upper part of the spine. In order to straighten the spine further pull up through the crown of the head so that the neck lengthens and you can feel a movement upwards along the entire length of the spine. Imagine there is an invisible string attached to the crown of your head gently extending straight up.

23

While practising your breathing, try and be aware of how your body feels. What parts of the body are rising and falling? Feel the breath passing through the nostrils with each inhalation and exhalation. Why is the in-breath cooler than the out-breath? Because you are inhaling air that has been at the temperature of the outside environment, and exhaling air that has been in the warm environment of your own body. Begin to understand the effect every breath is having on the body and mind.

ABDOMINAL BREATHING

There are three main types of breathing. The first is clavicular or chest breathing, which is the most common, but also the worst way of breathing. The shoulders and collarbone are raised while the stomach is contracted

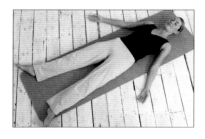

during inhalation. Lots of unconscious effort is made in this type of breathing, but a minimum amount of air is obtained. Intercostal breathing, or middle breathing, is the second type and involves the rib muscles expanding the ribcage. Although better than clavicular/chest breathing, it still does not introduce the maximum amount of air to your system. The third, and best type of breathing is abdominal breathing, or tummy breathing, because it brings air into the deepest and lowest parts of the lungs. Breathing in this way is slow and deep, and the diaphragm is properly used. Abdominal breathing is best done lying flat on the floor in the Corpse Pose (see page 36).

Place one hand on the abdomen. The ideal spot to put the hand is over the belly button. Now take a deep, slow breath using as much of the lower part of your stomach as possible. As you inhale, feel the abdomen rising and as you exhale feel the abdomen lower. Really feel your hand rise and fall as you breathe. Don't look at your stomach, keep your head flat on the floor. If you wish to see how much your stomach is rising and falling, place a few books on it so that you can keep your head flat but still see the movement.

Continue for a minute or so.

24

Initially you may find it strange to be using the stomach and your breathing may seem unnatural and make you feel tired. This is fine and is all part of learning. Like anything else, your body will react in funny ways to new ideas. Keep breathing and feel the air going deep down into your body. Gradually you will start to breathe like this all the time and you may even struggle to remember how you used to breathe! It is always a great pleasure to see students discovering how to breathe properly again and the benefits it brings.

FULL YOGIC BREATH

In the full yogic breath, inhalation and exhalation occur in three stages. First, the tummy is filled with air through the process of abdominal breathing. Then you inhale sideways into the ribcage, using the intercostal muscles to expand the ribcage and pull air into the middle part of the lungs. Lastly, air is inhaled into the upper part of the chest. The three types of breathing discussed at the beginning of this section, abdominal/tummy, intercostal/middle and clavicular/chest are all incorporated into the full yogic breath in order to gain the maximum benefits from each inhalation and exhalation.

Sit comfortably in a cross-legged position. Place cushions under the bottom if needed. The important thing is to be relaxed and comfortable, with the spine as straight as possible. If the back is very uncomfortable, try sitting against a wall, or upright on a chair. Place one hand on the abdomen and the other hand on the ribcage, just above the lower hand. Inhale slowly and deeply, feeling the abdomen expand as you inhale. Once the tummy is reasonably full of air, continue to inhale into the ribcage and then into the upper chest. Pause for just a moment and then begin your exhalation feeling your chest lowering, ribs closing and tummy releasing. If it doesn't happen in this order precisely that really is all right, the main thing is that your body is comfortable and not straining as you breathe out. As you exhale, the air will leave the lower lung first, then the middle, and then lastly the air will leave the upper lung. Always be relaxed, always keep your breathing at a steady pace and always try to be aware of everything that your body is telling you about your breath.

Practise this type of breathing on a regular basis. In time it will become easy. This is a great way to energize the body or to relax it during times of stress. It is another tool for your tool box and should be used at every opportunity. For example I love to do my breathing while I'm on public transport, it is a great way to pass the time! Practise for at least a couple of minutes each day.

ALTERNATE NOSTRIL BREATHING

There are many different techniques for alternate nostril breathing and the one I will show you is among the easiest. Why is this an important exercise? Have you ever noticed that you are generally able to breathe more easily through one nostril than the other? Or that you may be completely blocked up on one side, and then twenty minutes later it is the other nostril that is blocked? None of this should surprise us. The breath alternates between the right and left nostril roughly every fifty minutes in a healthy person. If you are unable to breathe through one nostril for over two hours it is considered to be a sign that illness is imminent. That so few of us are aware of this fact shows how little attention we pay to our breathing. Alternate nostril breathing tries to balance both nostrils and maintain equilibrium in the body, as well as for general cleansing of the whole body

Sit in a comfortable cross-legged position if you can or on a chair if you can't. Take your left hand and place it on your left knee. Take your right hand and fold the index and middle fingers down to the palm of the hand so that the thumb and two end fingers are straight, or make a fist and then straighten the thumb and two end fingers. Either way the first finger and the middle finger should be pressed down into the palm. Maintain this hand position throughout. Close the right nostril with the right thumb and inhale through the left nostril for four slow counts with a full yogic breath. Now, in one movement release the thumb from the right nostril while simultaneously using your two end fingers to block the left nostril. Exhale for eight slow counts. Once the exhalation is finished, inhale into your right nostril for four slow counts, then place the right thumb back onto the right nostril to block it and exhale slowly through the left nostril for eight slow counts. Repeat this for up to ten cycles at first, building up to any level you feel comfortable with. A short

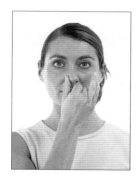
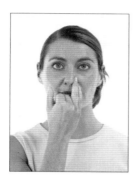
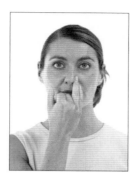
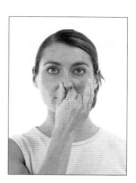

inhale   *exhale*   *inhale*   *exhale*

form of Alternate Nostril Breathing is: inhale left, exhale right, inhale right, exhale left. Don't feel you have to start with the counting I have suggested; if you are more comfortable starting with a smaller number of counts, go right ahead. This is breathing: there is no limit to how much you can do. If you begin to struggle due to one nostril being excessively blocked then stop and try again at a later time. As always, comfort is everything.

Try to practise your breathing techniques as much as possible to begin with. As your breathing improves you will find it easier to remain in the asanas comfortably for longer periods. You will probably find every sporting exercise you do will become easier and more comfortable. For something so vital to our life, we give very little time to understanding our breathing properly. Try it out, you may find that you have been doing it right all these years and can be pleased. However, you may also discover how little you knew about the inhalations and exhalations that keep you alive. It is the journey and the discovery that are important.

27

Mind Training

What was the last thought that you can remember crossing your mind? Chances are it probably wasn't too important. That's the way our minds work. Hundreds of thoughts fly by every day and how many of them do you think you will remember in a week? How about a year from now? So much chatter goes through our mind that we often have a hard time sifting through what we do or don't need. Our mind is our home; would you like to live every day in a messy, cluttered home?

It doesn't take any great skill or strength to learn to control the mind. Like anything else it just takes a bit of discipline and the desire to create more space to allow you to see life more clearly. At first it will only take five to ten minutes a day. But as for your yoga practice, the peace and happiness gained from slowing the mind down for a few minutes will grow, and soon you will find the benefits creeping into everything you do.

Have you ever calmed yourself down by breathing slowly and deeply? Well, you were using principles of mind control when you did that. The breath and the mind are tied together and observation of proper breathing forms the first foundation of mind control. By regulating and observing the breath you will begin to see what you always knew was happening, but couldn't quite explain! Thoughts will begin to slow down and you will find yourself simply observing their flow, without grasping at them or becoming attached to any of them.

As you continue on your journey of observation you will become aware of many different things. Your body might be stiff, or nervous, or maybe you will even be wonderfully relaxed. Our physical state constantly changes from day to day. Through regular practice of mind control, you will be aware of how the changes in your physical body are linked to changes in your mental state. Before too long, that increased awareness will manifest itself in everything you do. Awareness is the second foundation on which mind control is built.

Not many of you will be used to sitting completely still, doing nothing but breathing. It may feel strange to begin with. That is why concentration is the third foundation of mind control and, for beginners, is probably the most important. At first you may find your mind unable to settle into any kind of rhythm, and you will probably find yourself distracted by sounds, thoughts, smells and even sights if you open your eyes. Don't worry about it. This is an exercise in concentration and nobody is going to be perfect to begin with. Learn to focus yourself and stay fixed on a particular point; this will help you greatly.

The more you practise the more you begin to understand that there is no magic involved, no secret method and no quick way to mental peace. Instead, you simply find that slowly over time your mind begins to clear, your thoughts slow down, and you are much more in control of your emotions. When that starts happening, mind control becomes a joy. Those five minutes in the morning start turning into fifteen minutes, then twenty, and soon you find that even in the middle of a busy day you will make the time to just sit and breathe for a few moments, bringing the mind back home, where it is most comfortable.

To get you started, I have come up with three simple techniques to exercise your skills of observation, awareness and concentration. These are simple tools that may be done for five to ten minutes a day at first, preferably in the morning when you first get up. Why in the morning? Well, it's simply that after a good night's sleep your mind will probably be relatively clear and refreshed. Try the evening by all means, but it may be more difficult to relax and concentrate after a long and busy day. You should try and find the same time and spot to sit comfortably and practise each day. Familiarity relaxes the mind, and over time it will begin to see sitting in that spot for ten minutes as another part of the daily routine. Just make sure you are comfortable. Sitting cross-legged, with a folded cushion underneath your bottom will gently tilt the pelvis forward which helps to straighten the spine, but if that is uncomfortable then by all means use a chair. Just relax and enjoy it.

MIND-TRAINING TECHNIQUES

OBSERVATION

Sit in a comfortable position and try to straighten the back as much as possible, keeping the chin parallel to the floor so that you are looking directly forward. Place your hands comfortably on your knees or lower thighs. Close your eyes. For the next minute or so simply observe the breath. Don't try and change it, or influence it, simply watch the inhalation and exhalation just as they are. Next, and without any strain, start taking full, proper, deep abdominal breaths. Focus on bringing as much air into your body as possible, and then completely exhaling all the air all the way down to the bottom of your tummy. Repeat this ten times. Now bring your breath back to its natural state and observe whether it feels different to before you started abdominal breathing. Is it quicker or slower? Are your nostrils clearer than they were? There are no right or wrong answers, simply observe the breath. If thoughts enter your mind simply allow them to pass away and continue to observe the breath. If you do find that you have become tied up with a thought and drifted off, don't worry. Simply allow that thought to pass and come back to the breathing. Continue this sitting observation for up to five minutes or however long you are comfortable. Gradually you will find it easier to observe the breath throughout this period, without any thoughts distracting you. Enjoy the space you have created.

AWARENESS

Find a relaxed position to sit in, close your eyes and allow your breath to be natural and steady. Relax the entire body and mind, and for a minute or so simply be aware of how each part of the body feels. Always be aware of the breath. Now ask yourself, 'If I had one wish, and only one wish, anything at all I wanted in the entire world, what would it be?' Observe your mind coming up with its answers and be aware of each one. Ask yourself 'Why?' to each answer and see how your mind begins to change its answers. Simply be aware of this changing nature for up to five minutes. There is no right or wrong answer, it is simply a little game to help your awareness of how you think. It is different for every one of us.

This same exercise can be used, with only a slight variation, whenever you have a problem or a situation in your life which is causing you discomfort. Just sit down, relax the body, and observe the breath. Instead of asking yourself what wish you would make, tell yourself the problem clearly and slowly and ask, 'Why is this causing me discomfort?' Whatever your mind throws out as a reason ask 'Why?' again and just follow your mind as it leads you through the puzzle. Once again, this will not lead to instant satisfaction, but understanding the way your mind works is the first step to any kind of lasting mental peace and happiness.

CONCENTRATION

Whenever we begin mind control, the hardest thing is often just staying in the same spot for five or ten minutes. It sounds so easy but how many times in our lives, even when we are asleep, are we perfectly still for that length of time? At our desk we fidget and move around, while eating we shift our legs and wriggle our shoulders, on the train we shuffle our bottoms or turn the pages of our book. We are always moving! Concentration is vital to mind control, as it is for so many things we do. This exercise is ideal for improving our powers of concentration.

Find something on which you can concentrate for a long period. It could be a picture, or a statue, but best of all would be a candle flame. Place the object in front of you and sit comfortably, observing the natural breath. Look directly at the object and concentrate completely on it, trying not to blink without forcing your eyes to stay open. Focus on every part of the object, the different colours, shapes and outlines. After about a minute of this, close your eyes and try to imagine the object you were looking at forming in the blackness in front of your closed eyes. Simply relax and see how much of the object re-creates itself on your personal movie screen. After about a minute open your eyes again and concentrate on the object for another minute. Try to find the gaps in your mental picture and see what is actually there. Concentrate on every part of the object, and after another minute close your eyes again and try to create the image in front of your closed eyes. Repeat up to three times.

Gradually you will find that you are able to concentrate longer without blinking, and that the picture formed in front of your closed eyes will become clearer and clearer and will stay imprinted on your mind for more time. You will also find your concentration improves generally in your daily life.

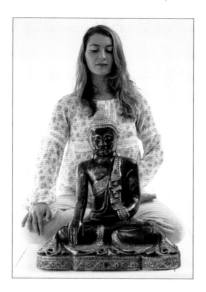

AND THEN?

Well, you have learned the first basic tools of meditation. I personally prefer calling this mind control because meditation can sound too serious and daunting. But they are the same thing and you shouldn't be afraid of the word meditation. There are many other tools to help mind control, just as there are many tools of yoga. In fact, mind control is a huge part of yoga itself and so when you are doing your daily mind control, you are also doing your yoga. Please don't put pressure on yourself to get huge results. Mind control is just about slowing down and finding space. You will see the benefits eventually, and when you do you won't want to stop, believe me! On days when I have had to miss my own mind-training practice, I can feel that something is not quite right. It can be simply a great way of calming down the chatter in your head and finding one voice you are comfortable listening to.

Relaxation

The art of proper relaxation is central to yoga. Learning to relax properly is every bit as important as learning to perform the asanas correctly.

What comes to your mind when you think of relaxation? To most of us, images of sitting in front of the television, taking a long stroll or going on holiday. But to truly relax is so much more than just non-movement or the absence of daily stress. When we watch television our senses are subject to a constant barrage of images, sounds and ideas that stop our mind from properly relaxing. A nice stroll may relax the mind to an extent, but of course our bodies are still functioning and burning up energy through movement. And how many times have you found that the long-awaited holiday was actually just as stressful as life at home or at work? True relaxation brings peace to the body and mind, allowing us to rest in the pulse of the universe, grounded and yet alert and aware of events around us. If the asanas are tools to energize and invigorate, then proper relaxation is a tool to cool down and balance the system.

From the moment we wake up we put our body and mind under strain. This strain continues throughout the day, and seldom stops until we finally get back into bed and shut down our system for the night. Even during sleep however, tensions built up during the day still affect the way we rest and recuperate.

Every physical action creates tension in our muscles. On many occasions we are able to observe this tension, whether it is because of extreme physical exertion, or simply due to a long day of sitting at a desk in front of a computer with our back curled forward and shoulders hunched. Most of us have come to accept this tension as a natural part of our lives, and have forgotten what it feels like to let go and simply exist without any physical effort. Indeed, many of us may actually have convinced ourselves that we perform our daily routines better in a state of tension, as if tightness and strain actually assist, rather than hinder, our efforts. This is not the case. Any performer or athlete will confirm that at their best, an unconscious relaxation of the body naturally takes place, allowing them to perform their job efficiently and to the best of their ability. Proper relaxation is a gift every one of us should give to our bodies each and every day, and is something that may be learned and enjoyed by anyone.

Equally, tension is also a factor for our minds, and is caused by emotions, such as anger, sorrow, greed, envy, hatred and anxiety. We all have these emotions. How many of us can say truthfully that we are able to keep them under control at all times? Uncontrolled emotion uses up just as much energy as physical activity, although we are seldom aware of this fact. Picture in your mind a person reacting with anger. See the tension and strain throughout the entire body: the clenched fists, the mad eyes, the heavy breathing. Now ask yourself whether a single part of the body or mind is inactive during that moment? Anger is probably the most obvious emotion, but you can probably see how every emotion leads to our body and mind using energy that should be going towards keeping us healthy and free from disease. As the energy, or prana, which our system requires to keep us functioning at peak efficiency slowly dissipates under the tensions of our body and mind, mental fatigue increases, resulting in additional strain on our muscles and internal organs. Proper relaxation is about letting go of the emotions, observing them for what they are and understanding their changing nature.

In yoga the asanas are used to create additional energy for our system. Proper relaxation seals this energy, cares for it and provides a space for it to flow throughout every part of our existence. As you spend more and more time in proper relaxation, you will become aware of just how tense you previously were, and what true relaxation should feel like.

35

RELAXATION TECHNIQUES

THE CORPSE POSE

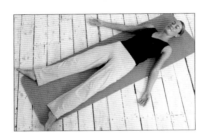

The Corpse Pose requires you to lie flat on the floor, completely relaxed, simply breathing. Sounds easy, doesn't it? It is surprising how many people feel uncomfortable in this posture due to the fact that they are unable to relax and just let go. Relaxation before, during and after any physical exercise is vital in order to bring your heartbeat back to normal, circulate fresh air and energy through your body, eliminate lactic acid from your muscles, and to calm you mentally. The Corpse Pose is the best position for all these wonderfully refreshing things to happen. The technique is very easy but, like all yoga, it requires you to be present and aware of your entire body and mind in order for the full benefits to be felt.

36

The Technique

① Lie down completely flat on the floor, with your eyes looking straight up and your chin tucked slightly towards your throat so that it is at a 90° angle to the floor. It is vital that the head stays straight and does not twist from side to side.

② Straighten your legs and separate them so they are about a metre apart with the toes relaxed and falling out to the sides.

> *Note:* For those who have bad backs and find lying flat with straight legs to be uncomfortable, you can bend the knees and place the soles of your feet flat on the floor. This relieves some pressure on the lower back.

③ Place your arms flat and away from the body at about a 45° angle, and turn your palms up to face the ceiling. Relax your arms, fingers and shoulders.

④ Think about your entire spine relaxing towards the floor, including the back of your neck and your lower back, which may be slightly raised from the floor to begin with.

⑤ Close your eyes. Focus on breathing naturally through the nose, being aware of how it feels to breath in this position.

As mentioned above, the Corpse Pose should be done before you practise yoga, whenever you feel your body needs it during your practice, and also as a way to relax your body after all postures have been completed.

INITIAL RELAXATION
To be done prior to exercising.

Lie flat in the Corpse Pose and be aware of your breathing. How does it feel? Mentally check every part of your body. Are there any aches and pains that may hinder your yoga practice? If so, imagine your breathing to be sending energy directly to those parts of your body that may be feeling tense or uncomfortable. Constantly return to the breathing and allow it to relax your body and mind. Inhale energy into and through your body, exhale and breathe out tension with each breath. Let go of any worries you may have, try and forget about them until your yoga practice is over. Just relax and give the next twenty or thirty minutes, or however long you wish to practise, to yourself. This is your time so make the most of it. Stay in this position for a few minutes until you feel fully relaxed.

37

RELAXATION BETWEEN ASANAS

When you feel that your body and mind need to rest, listen to them. Often, when you have been working on a challenging asana you will want to rest so do return to a state of deep relaxation and examine what affect the asana has had on your body and breath. Use this time to balance all the energy in the body and return to a comfortable state. Do not begin your next asana until your breath has returned to normal and your body feels relaxed and energized by a fresh intake of oxygen and energy.

In the Basic Postures section I have often indicated which pose is best for relaxation following the more challenging asanas, but you can chose the one that feels most comfortable. The three are:

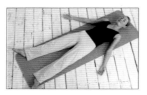

Corpse Pose

(see page 36)

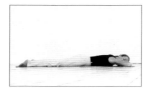

Lying on Front

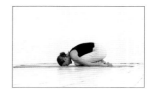

Child's Pose

(see page 61)

FINAL RELAXATION

Too many of us finish any type of physical exercise without properly bringing the body and mind back to a rested and comfortable state. We just carry on with our day without allowing the full benefits of our exercise to sink in and circulate through the body. Final relaxation is vital and at least five minutes (ideally ten minutes if you were practising for an hour or more) is necessary to scan your body and mind and ensure that you have relaxed every part of them. There are two main types of relaxation: physical and mental. Each brings its own benefits and they should be practised one after another.

PHYSICAL RELAXATION

Since it is often hard initially for beginners to relax, it is important that you understand what it feels like for the body to be tense. This often allows the beginner to relax further than they may have thought possible.

This is usually the final relaxation. Lie in the Corpse Pose and breathe steadily. You are going to tense and relax various parts of the body gradually, but always remember to breathe through the nose and be aware of what your body is telling you.

①   Inhale and raise the right leg 5 cm from the floor. Tense the right leg, feel the tightness through your whole leg. After 3 to 5 seconds of tensing, exhale and relax the right leg and allow it to drop to the floor by itself. If dropping your leg like this is at all uncomfortable, it may mean you lifted your leg higher than 5 cm. Repeat with your left leg.

②   Inhale and raise the hips 5 cm from the floor, pressing down through your heels and lifting the groin area towards the ceiling. Tense the buttocks and backs of the legs. This is a wonderful stretch but can be uncomfortable for beginners, so take it easy! Hold the tension for 3 to 5 seconds and then exhale and relax completely and allow the hips to fall back to the floor.

③   Inhale and raise the chest off the floor, tense the upper body and feel your shoulder blades coming closer together behind your back. Relax and gently drop the chest to the floor.

④   Inhale and raise the right arm 5 cm from the floor. Tense the entire arm. Clench your fist; now extend your fingers as much as possible. Exhale, release and let the arm fall gently to the floor. Repeat with the left arm.

⑤   Inhale and raise the shoulders towards the ears, tense and relax. Drop the shoulders towards your feet, tense and relax.

⑥   Scrunch up your entire face. Tense every part of your jaw, cheeks, eyes, ears and forehead. Imagine you are turning your face into a dried prune! Now relax everything.

⑦   Tilt your head slightly back, open your eyes and mouth as wide as possible, let your tongue hang out (try and touch your chin with your tongue), and silently let out a large exhalation.

Now just relax and be aware of how the entire body feels. Take a few moments to check each part, creating a mental checklist that you can go through each time you relax.

MENTAL RELAXATION

40

Now that we have tensed and relaxed each part of the body you are ready to use auto-suggestion to further relax and centre yourself. Take your time with this one, the mind has a habit of wandering at first. Just stay with it for a few more minutes – you will enjoy the benefits for hours if you do.

①   Beginning with the toes feel as if a wave of relaxation is sweeping over your entire body. Use the breath to imagine clean air and energy coming into your body with every inhalation. On the exhalation concentrate on releasing negative energy or physical blockages. Mentally relax each toe, telling yourself slowly as you breathe out, 'I am relaxing my toes, I am relaxing my toes, my toes are relaxed.' Focus on that part of your body and feel it relaxing.

②   Now proceed to your feet and ankles. Feel the relaxation sweeping through these areas. Take as much time as you need. Always use the exhalation to tell your body to relax. Inhale energy, exhale tension.

③   Exhale and feel the relaxation moving up the legs, relaxing the calves, the knees, and the thighs. Repeat the relaxation command for each part of the leg and be aware of how each area feels as tension is gradually released.

④   Exhale and relax the buttocks and feel the tension releasing from your lower back. Take time to concentrate on the back. This is very important because your back is under so much strain throughout the day. Give it this moment to relax properly. Feel the lower back begin to sink into the floor.

⑤   Feel the relaxation proceeding to your chest. Breathe very slowly and gently. Feel the chest and torso softening.

⑥   Bring your attention to the fingers and on an exhalation keep repeating the relaxation command to yourself, quietly and patiently, always using your breathing to pace yourself.

⑦   Slowly come up through the wrists, arms, elbows and shoulders. The shoulders are another place to focus your attention closely. As with the lower back, feel the shoulders relaxing into the floor. You should feel as though you could drop through to the centre of the earth if the floor weren't there to stop you.

⑧   Exhale and relax the neck, the jaw, the chin and cheeks, the mouth, the eyes and the forehead. Imagine your entire face melting, especially the cheeks softening, eyes resting and jaw releasing. Our faces hold an enormous amount of nervous tension and you should feel this tension disappearing.

⑨   Now breathe out between the eyebrows. I find this helps me feel my mind is resting and creating space there. Just relax and observe how your body feels right now. Take a few moments, or however long you need, just to rest in this position and feel the normal state of your breath.

⑩   Now give yourself a big thank you for taking this time to observe your body and mind!!!

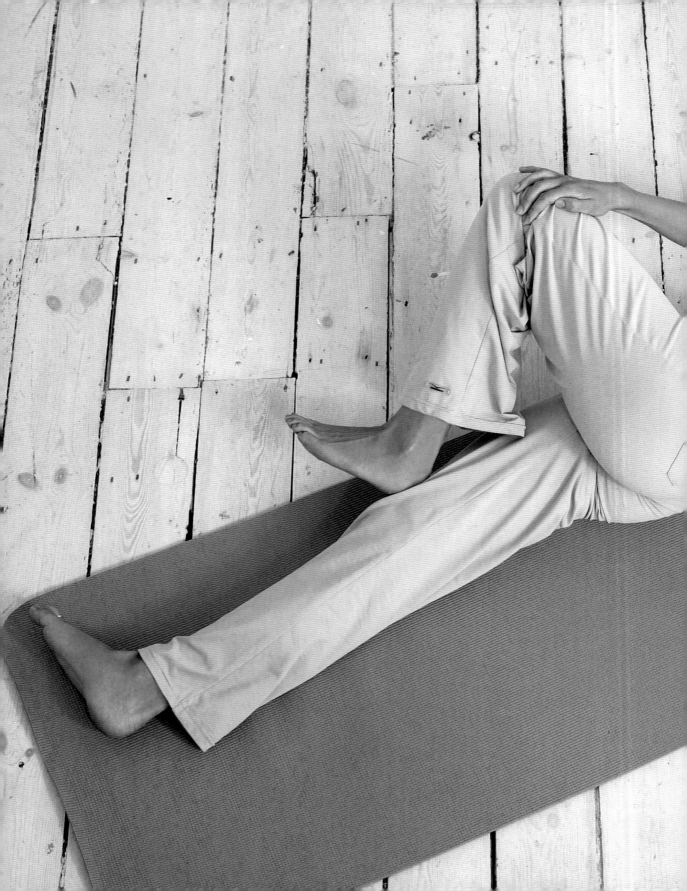

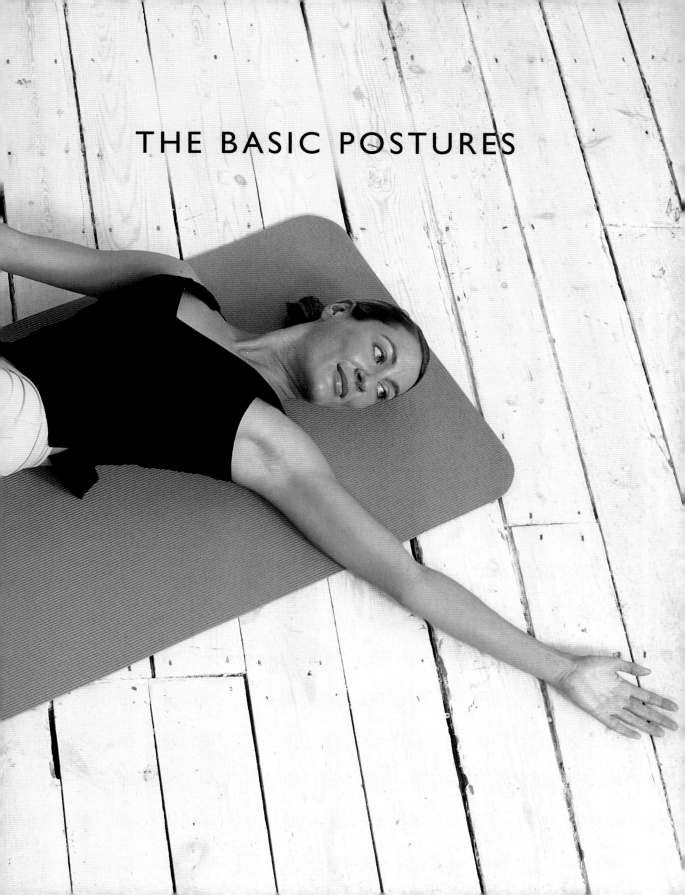

THE BASIC POSTURES

The Lying Sequence

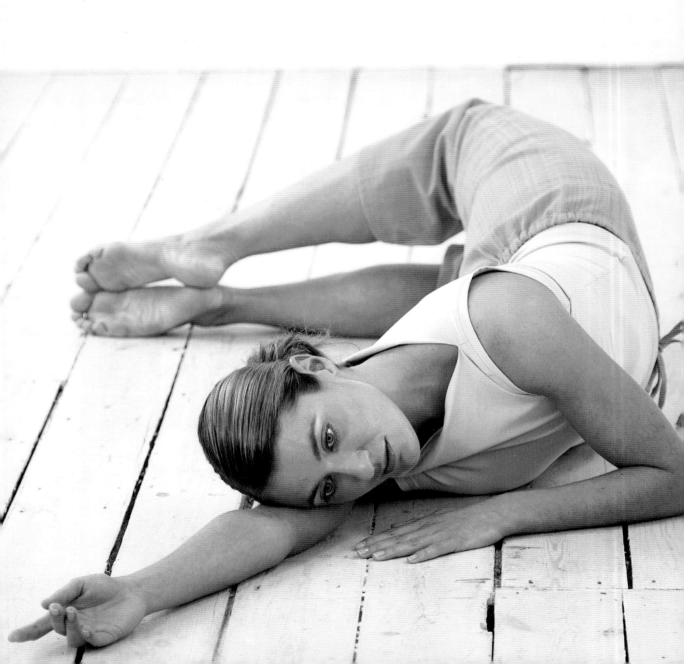

Now you're ready to begin. The postures in the lying, sitting and standing sequences were chosen to give you a complete yoga class. Once you are familiar with the postures you should move smoothly from one to the next, focusing on the breath. Always stop and relax if your body needs to, but try to keep a continuous flow of movement. On page 92 the full programme is listed.

RELAXATION

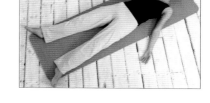

①   Lie in the Corpse Pose (see page 36) flat on your back, looking straight up. Have your legs about a metre apart. Allow your toes to fall outwards naturally. Take your arms a comfortable distance away from your body and turn your palms up. Think about your shoulders and lower back releasing down to the floor. Close your eyes and begin to breathe through your nose, slowly and easily.

②   Observe your natural breath. Be aware of how it feels today, right at this moment. After a while, slow it down by taking full deep yogic breaths. As you breathe be aware of your tummy, ribcage and finally your chest expanding with the inhalation and then contracting with the exhalation (see page 25 for a full explanation of full yogic breathing).

③   After a few minutes allow your breathing to return to its usual state. Observe each part of your body now. Do a small mental checklist of any aches and pains. How might they affect your yoga today? Be aware of your body and what it is telling you.

④   Now observe your mind. See if it is staying easily with the breath today. Often I find that when I first begin my practice my mind bounces from one thing to another, so I try and keep my thoughts on my breath – how it feels, how long I can breathe in and out. Although I try to stay focused on my breath, my mind does wander, especially if I have had a busy day. All I can do is gently coax it back each time and little by little the mind slows and gradually it becomes easier to concentrate on the breath.

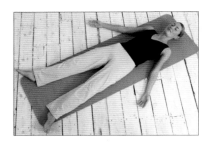

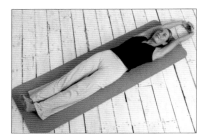

BIG STRETCH

Lie flat on your back in the Corpse Pose. Breathe through the nostrils slowly and relax the body.

①   Inhale and stretch your arms outwards and backwards so they circle round and meet behind your head as close to the floor as possible. Try and keep your arms on the floor throughout the movement. If your shoulders are stiff this may not be possible, so just think about keeping your arms low. If you can, interlock your fingers when your hands meet behind your head.

②   Inhale and stretch your arms away from you towards the wall behind you. Keep the hands as low as possible and feel the entire upper body stretch. Feel the spine lengthening and awakening. Think about your lower back relaxing and moving towards the floor. Always remember to keep breathing. After a few seconds relax the stretch.

③   Bring the legs together, flex the feet, then point the toes away from you.

④   Now bring your entire body into the stretch on the next inhalation. Don't wonder if you are doing it right, YOU ARE!!! This is your body, listen to what it is telling you and be aware of what it needs. Keep breathing. Even though you are stretching you never tense the body. Try to stay as relaxed as possible.

⑤   Stay in this posture for as long as is comfortable to begin with. Often our bodies are not used to this type of stretch and you may feel cramp in the feet and toes, or tightness in the shoulders and upper back. This is your body telling you it has had enough, listen to it. It will get better over time.

Benefits
✓ Elongates and stretches the spine and the waist.
✓ Shoulders rotate and open.
✓ Space is created enabling you to breathe more deeply.

Mistakes
✗ The feet are allowed to wander.
✗ Don't worry if the hands won't meet behind the head, it will happen eventually.

General Warning
❗ If you have any back pain whatsoever it may be a good idea to bend the knees slightly when in this stretch.

THE BALL

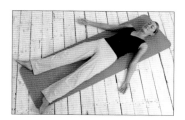

Lie flat on your back in the Corpse Pose. Breathe through the nostrils slowly and relax the body.

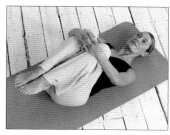

① Exhale and draw both your knees towards your chest, knees close together, feet off the floor. Hold the knees, or whichever part of your legs is comfortable. If you find this uncomfortable, open the knees a bit.

② With each exhalation bring the knees a bit closer towards the chest, feeling the lower back releasing as you gradually apply more downward pressure. As always, this downward pressure should only be as much as is comfortable. While in the posture think about sending the tailbone, the lowest vertebra of the spine, downwards while at the same time lengthening it away from the body. As you do this you will also feel a stretch in the back of your legs. Keep the breath going and relax slightly with each inhalation.

③ If the back is feeling particularly stiff, it can sometimes be great to rock gently from side to side – not too much – which massages the entire back. Imagine your back is a piece of pastry that you are trying to roll out as you rock. Focus on the areas that feel tense or tired and massage those feelings away.

④ Stay in this position for about 5 to 10 rounds of very slow rhythmic breathing, but always pay attention to how your back is feeling. This is a great posture to release the spine, but it can be very demanding at first.

Benefits
✓ It releases the spine.
✓ Excellent for relieving stiff backs/hamstrings/hips and for improving general flexibility.

Mistakes
✗ Make sure that the lower back does not over-arch in transition from the relaxation position to a ball position.
✗ The lower back is allowed to come off the floor.
✗ The shoulders and neck leave the floor.

General Warning
❗ If you have a weakness in the back then take one leg at a time into the ball.

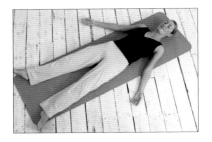

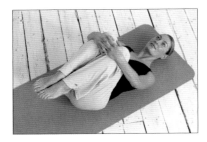

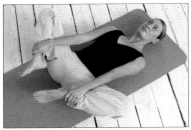

THE FROG

Lie flat on your back in the Corpse Pose. Breathe through the nostrils slowly and relax the body.

① Keep the breath going steadily throughout. Bring the knees towards the chest and open them leaving the heels together. Put your arms through the middle of your legs and hold on to your shins, knees, ankles or feet — whichever suits you best (you are aiming to hold the ankles comfortably).

② Stay in this position for 3 to 6 rounds of very slow breathing.

③ Feel the exhalation moving to areas that might feel stiff and try to dissolve any tension in the body through the act of exhaling. Be aware of the pressure on the knees in this posture. Feel them dropping out to the sides and the feet coming closer towards the face. If you have any discomfort, focus the breath down into that area; this is just a sign that the body is stretching naturally.

④ Make sure to keep the neck relaxed and feel it sinking down into the floor. Keep the chin slightly tilted towards the chest so that the back of the neck is stretched as well.

⑤ Be aware of the lower back. Relax it with every breath and try and keep the bottom flat on the floor.

Benefits
- ✓ Excellent for opening the hips and keeping the hip joint supple and healthy.
- ✓ Improves the flexibility of the ankles.
- ✓ Tones the inside of the thighs.

Mistakes
- ✗ The lower back leaves the floor.
- ✗ The shoulders and neck leave the floor.

General Warning
- ❗ Be very cautious if you have had back or hip problems.

ANKLE CIRCLES

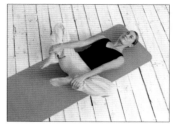

Lie on your back in the Frog.

①   Try and hold the ankles. If you can't, place your palms on your knees.

②   Allow the feet to be about 30 cm or so apart and circle your feet in opposite directions. Think about creating large, juicy circles with your feet. Do about 3 to 6 slow, big circles and then change direction and circle the other way. Keep breathing.

③   After circling the ankles in both directions, bring your knees back together and fold them towards your chest. Now rest your hands on the knees and relax the body. Observe how your ankles, groin, lower back and hamstrings feel.

Benefits

✓ The ankles are massaged and flexibility is increased.

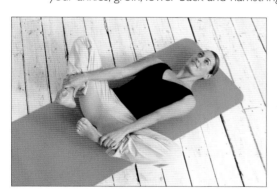
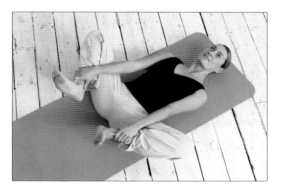
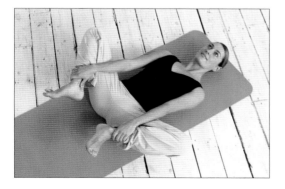
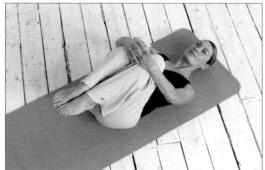

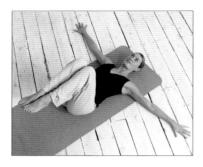

DOUBLE KNEE SPINAL TWIST

Lie flat on your back and bring your knees into the chest, feet off the floor, lower back relaxed and lengthened, so you are in a ball.

① Make sure the knees are together, the sides of the feet touching and off the floor. Spread the arms out to each side along the floor at shoulder height, with the palms flat to the floor. Spread your fingers out, imagining you have sunshine in your palms and the sun is extending out of your fingers. Think of your shoulders relaxing and sinking.

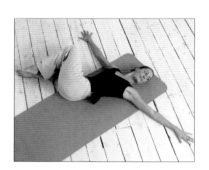

② Inhale fully but gently. On the exhalation take both knees together over to the right. Try to move slowly and calmly. Feel the arms, hands and shoulders pressing into the floor as your torso twists. You are trying to keep both shoulders and arms on the floor but, often, beginners find that their opposite shoulder and arm do come up slightly and, of course, this is fine. Keep going until your right knee and right foot are resting on the floor with your left leg lying on top of it.

③ Turn your head in the opposite direction to your legs and look at your outstretched left arm. If your left shoulder and arm are off the floor, think of relaxing in that area and feel the natural downward pressure of gravity working on your arm – use your exhalation to help with this. Gradually work towards having both palms flat on the floor throughout this posture.

④ Stay here for 3 to 6 rounds of slow breathing. When in this posture think about sending the breath across the collarbones and along each arm and hand to help release tension that you may be holding. Always think about relaxing and lengthening the spine in any twist.

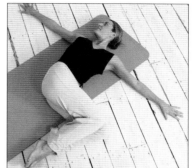

⑤   To come out of the twist inhale and bring your knees
      and legs back to centre. Make sure you press your arms,
      palms and shoulders into the floor as you come back.
      Really use the floor (try pulling in your tummy muscles,
      this will help). Then exhale and move your legs over to
      the left-hand side and repeat. Keep the knees together
      at all times.

⑥   For a more advanced version, hold the knees and feet a
      few inches off the floor when you have brought them
      over. You can also try speeding up the movements so that you move to one
      side or the other with every breath, always pausing with the knees and feet
      slightly raised, before beginning again. If you do this, remember that you exhale
      when taking the legs down towards the floor and inhale to bring them back
      to the centre.

⑦   When you've finished, bring the knees back in front of you then gently bring
      them towards the chest. Put the feet on the floor, relax and think of your
      palms, arms and shoulders melting into the floor.

Benefits
✔ Tiredness and tightness relieved, especially in the lower back.
✔ Pelvic and abdominal organs are toned through the massaging action of the twist.
✔ Rectifies disorders of the hip joint, excellent for people who sit for long periods.
✔ Stimulates the nervous system.
✔ Improves digestion and eliminates constipation by stretching the tummy muscles and internal organs.
✔ Helps keep the spine mobile through rotation.

Mistakes
✘ Arms and hands not pressing down into the floor.
✘ The opposite shoulder to the rotation lifts from the floor too much.
✘ The legs and knees allowed to separate. Keep them together.
✘ Holding the breath. Just because you are twisting, don't stop breathing.

General Warning
❗ If you have problems with your lower back then please do this posture with the feet on the floor throughout the whole sequence.

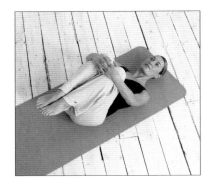

HAMSTRING STRETCHES

Lie flat on your back, knees bent, feet off the floor. Place your hands on your knees and allow the weight of your hands and arms to press the knees further towards the chest. Relax and feel the spine lengthen.

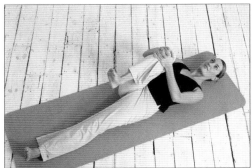

① Place both hands on top of the right knee and on an exhalation straighten out the left leg until the heel touches the floor. Stretch through the left heel so that the entire left leg comes down towards the floor. Throughout this posture keep straightening and lengthening the leg, gradually pressing it down into the floor more and more. Slowly bring your right knee further in towards your chest and keep the tailbone pressing down and away. Try not to turn your hips in any way, keep them straight. Keep your neck relaxed and lengthened.

② You will now go into a hamstring release which can often be quite a stretch, so be careful. If you cannot straighten your right leg immediately, don't worry. However, that is the eventual goal so think about straightening and lengthening up through the heel constantly as you practise this posture. On an exhalation straighten the right leg upwards, driving your heel towards the ceiling. Hold your leg with both hands wherever is comfortable, but don't hold on directly behind the knee because this puts a huge amount of strain on the knee and can lead to injury. If you cannot hold the calf then just hold the back of the thigh. More flexibility will come in time. Don't forget about the left leg!!

③ With each exhalation think of straightening the right leg and with each inhalation imagine the knee softening. Your breathing will definitely help, so really focus on the breath. Remember to take it easy, the leg should never shake with tension. Approach this slowly and you will eventually see the results.

④ To finish, draw the right leg back to your chest and relax it. Then bend the left leg up and bring the knees together, with your hands on top of them. Think about lengthening the spine and breathe slowly.

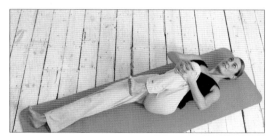 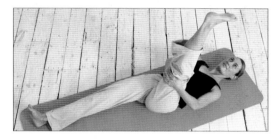

⑤ Repeat the exercise on the other side.

⑥ Hold this posture as long as is comfortable for you.

⑦ If you find it really uncomfortable you could try putting a belt over the raised foot and holding an end in each hand. This also assists the upper body to stay relaxed.

Benefits
✓ The hamstring stretches and lengthens.
✓ The hips loosen.
✓ The backs of the legs and the lower back are stretched and massaged.

Mistakes
✗ Be careful not to stretch the hamstrings too much. No strain.
✗ The body can be too tense; stay relaxed.
✗ The leg extended along the floor has a tendency to bend, try not to let this happen. Keep the working leg straight and drive through the heel.

General Warning
❗ Anyone with sciatica, a slipped disc or high blood pressure should be careful.

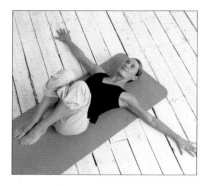

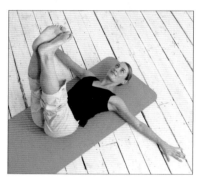

DOUBLE LEG STRETCH

Lie flat on the back, knees bent and pressed down towards the chest, feet off the floor. The arms should be stretched out to the sides at shoulder height with the palms and fingers spread out and pressed into the floor.

①   Keeping the palms flat to the floor, exhale and stretch your legs up to the ceiling. Flex your feet so that your toes are stretching down towards your head, heels driving upwards. Soften your knees and think of straightening the legs completely. How high your legs are is less important than keeping them straight. Be aware of your lower back while your legs straighten and think of the buttocks remaining firmly in contact with the floor.

②   Inhale, relax and bend the knees again, returning to the starting position. Repeat this movement slowly anywhere from 8 to 16 times until you feel the hips, thighs and hamstring warm up.

③   Always think about softening the knees and lengthening the legs. Feel the hamstrings stretch as you press the tailbone down towards the floor and outwards away from the head.

④   For an additional sequence just reverse the breath and straighten the legs on an inhalation, and exhale to return the legs to a bent position. As I said, don't worry about the height of the legs; this is all about straightening them fully.

Benefits
- ✓ Strengthens and massages the tummy and the internal organs.
- ✓ Warms up the hips, thighs and knees.
- ✓ Lengthens and stretches the hamstrings.

Mistakes
- ✗ Make sure that the lower back does not arch.
- ✗ Allowing the legs to bend in an attempt to get them higher.
- ✗ The arms and/or the hands lift from the floor.

General Warning
- ❗ Be careful if you have any knee or hip problems.

SINGLE LEG SPINAL TWIST

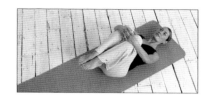

Lie flat on your back, knees bent towards the chest, feet off the floor. Place your hands on your knees and allow the weight of your hands and arms to press the knees towards the chest. Relax and feel the spine lengthen.

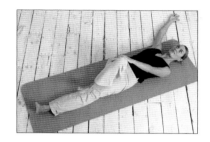

① Straighten your left leg out along the floor, feeling the buttocks press into the floor and the heel pull away. Place the right heel on the left leg just above the kneecap.

② Place the left hand on top of your right kneecap. Have your right arm along the floor at a slight diagonal going away from the right ear, with the palm up. If your right arm won't stay flat, that's okay, just keep letting gravity do its work and it will get there eventually.

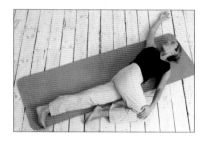

③ Slowly inhale. As you gently exhale take the left hand and guide the right leg along the floor on your left side. Allow the right hip to come off the floor as your body twists. At first you will probably find your right shoulder also comes off the floor. The aim is eventually to have both the right knee and the right shoulder flat on the floor. Think of opening the body into a diagonal line from the fingers of that outstretched right hand to the right

Benefits and Mistakes
✓✗ Same as for the Double Knee Spinal Twist (see page 51).

knee. Don't worry if you hear the occasional bone popping, that is totally normal, your spine is just realigning itself.

④ When you are in this posture try and relax as much as possible, using the exhalation to soften and relax the shoulders and letting your body sink into the spiral it has created. Always think of lengthening the spine.

⑤ Stay here for 3 to 6 long, deep breaths. Then bring the right knee back to the chest and bend the left leg again. Bring the knees together on an inhalation, and on the next inhalation straighten the right leg and repeat the twist to the other side, with the right hand leading the left leg down to the floor.

THE BRIDGE

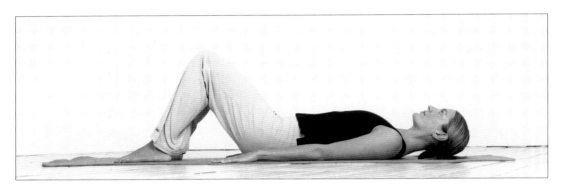

Lie flat on your back, knees bent, with the soles of the feet flat on the floor reasonably close to the buttocks. The feet should be about hip-width apart (take a hip width from the hip bones, not the outside of your hips), and the buttocks should be relaxed and flat on the floor. Place the arms close by the side of your body, palms flat on the floor, fingers relaxed and pointing towards the toes. Breathe and think of the neck and lower back sinking into the floor.

① Inhale deeply and, on the exhalation, tilt your pubic bone up towards your navel, rolling the tailbone up from the floor. Pressing down through the arms and the palms, begin rolling your spine off the floor, vertebra by vertebra, until

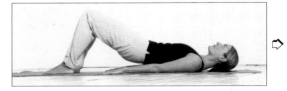 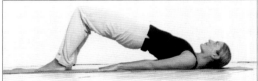

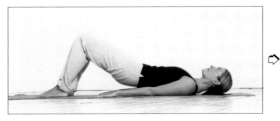 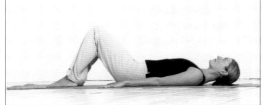

your knees, hips and shoulders are in line with each other. Hold the posture and make sure to keep the breath flowing.

② While you hold the posture think of extending the energy out through the knees. Imagine you have invisible strings attached to them gently pulling the knees and thighs away from you. Press down through your feet and palms and feel the shoulders keeping in contact with the floor. Open the chest and feel your collarbones curve upward to echo the shape of a smile. Keep the chin tilted slightly towards the chest so that the back of the neck remains extended. Try and imagine your belly button going up towards the ceiling. Hold the posture for one long deep breath.

③ Inhale and then exhale, and roll back in this order: soften and lower the chest first, then the ribs, then the lower back. You should try and return the spine to the floor vertebra by vertebra, taking your time and keeping the pubic bone tilted toward the navel until the entire spine is back on the floor.

④ If you want to increase the intensity of this posture simply hold yourself up in the Bridge for longer. If you do this, make sure to breathe slowly, don't allow your knees to drift apart, keep your feet and legs hip-width apart and keep pushing your navel towards the ceiling (i.e. don't let your tailbone drop).

Benefits
- ✓ The thyroid gland is stimulated.
- ✓ It realigns the spine, keeps it mobile and healthy.
- ✓ It's great for the shoulders and for relieving any backache.
- ✓ It massages and stretches the colon, improving digestion.
- ✓ It tones the female reproductive organs.
- ✓ It tones the buttocks.

Mistakes
- ✗ Having the legs further than hip-width apart.
- ✗ The feet roll over. Keep the weight evenly distributed between the feet, and the soles of the feet flat on the floor.
- ✗ Do not allow the head to tilt to either side. Keep it straight.
- ✗ The hips are allowed to drop down to floor. Keep pushing the navel towards the ceiling.

General Warning
- ❗ If you have a hernia or back or hip problems please take extreme care.

PREPARATION FOR AND FULL COBRA

Lie flat on your stomach. The legs and feet are together, the tops of the feet are flat on the floor. The arms are straight alongside the body with the palms down. The forehead is flat on the floor.

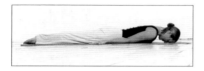

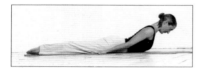

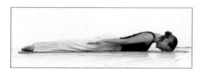

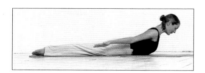

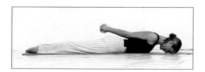

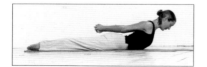

①   Inhale and extend your spine forward and up so that you lift your head and chest, and possibly even the ribs, from the floor. Open the chest widely by feeling your shoulder blades move together and back. Press the palms into the floor.

②   Exhale and extend the upper body slowly forward and down, in time with the exhalation.

③   Repeat 3 to 6 times focusing on feeling the tummy and the groin pressing into the floor and keeping the feet together and pressing down as well.

④   Now, here is the same sequence but with a slight variation. As you inhale and lengthen the spine forwards, lift your hands and arms off the floor as your head and chest rise. Make sure your arms don't hover any higher than a few centimetres. Repeat this 3 to 6 times focusing on these small movements and feeling, as a result, the lower back and thighs moving further into the floor.

⑤   Now take the hands and interlock them together behind your back. As you inhale and lengthen forward, think of trying to touch your heels with your hands. As your head and chest lift you will feel the chest open and the lower back press down. Don't poke your chin forwards. Keep your face looking down at the floor in front of you. Relax your neck and release any tension there. Repeat 3 to 6 times.

⑥   Finally it is time for the Full Cobra. Place the hands flat

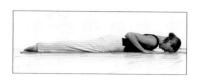

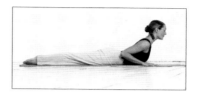

on the floor under the shoulders so that the fingertips are just in line with the top of your shoulders. Tuck your elbows in towards the body. Inhale and extend the head forward and up. Lengthen the spine forward and up and feel the chest rising from the floor. When you are almost at the point where you cannot go higher begin to apply pressure through the palms down into the floor. Keep opening the chest by pulling your shoulders back and down, while remembering to keep the elbows tucked in. Be careful the shoulders don't pop up towards the ears, keep them moving down and keep the shoulder blades coming together. Don't allow your elbows to lock and keep a slight bend in the arms.

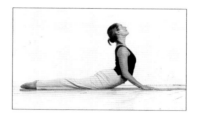

⑦ Exhale, roll the body down slowly, taking the pressure off the palms and allowing first the tummy, then chest, chin, and finally the forehead to rest on the floor. Relax and repeat.

⑧ If you ever feel any strain in the lower back come out of the posture immediately and rest, perhaps in Child's Pose (see page 61). Try again another day, there is no rush. Over time you will feel able to stay in the Full Cobra for longer and longer periods. Build up slowly and make sure your breathing is constant and natural. If your arms ever start shaking then come down; that is the body saying, 'enough'.

Benefits
✓ The front of the body is completely stretched.
✓ It massages the stomach, liver and kidneys.
✓ It helps regulate the thyroid gland.
✓ It strengthens the back, and over time pushes the spinal discs into correct alignment.
✓ It increases circulation in the back and tones the nerves.
✓ It tones the ovaries and the uterus and helps alleviate period problems.
✓ It stimulates the appetite and helps rid you of constipation.

Mistakes
✗ The elbows are straight. Keep them bent slightly.
✗ The feet are apart.
✗ The groin/pelvis is lifted from the floor.
✗ Using the arms too much instead of the body.
✗ Shoulders are up round the ears and are tense.

General Warning
❢ Take great care if you have a bad back.

THE EXTENDED CAT AND MOVING FROM THE COBRA TO THE CHILD'S POSE

This is a movement which takes us from the last posture into our preferred relaxation pose, the Child's Pose, to end the lying sequence. Luckily the movement incorporates a great stretch in itself – the Extended Cat.

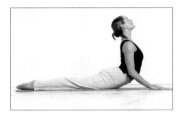

①   Come up into your Full Cobra and, in one movement, use your arms to push yourself away from the floor, lifting the stomach and hips. You should end up on all fours, with your knees and hands on the floor. Then take a big stretch backwards, taking your buttocks down as far as you can towards your heels, keeping the palms flat on the floor and the arms lengthened forwards. Stretch!

②   As you are in this stretch, feel the buttocks pressing down towards the heels and concentrate on relaxing the shoulders. This will allow your neck to relax and the forehead to sink towards the floor. Don't push down, allow gravity to do its own work.

③   Take your arms back alongside your body. This is the Child's Pose. Relax your shoulders and prepare for the final relaxation in the lying sequence.

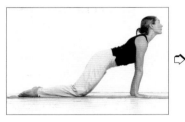 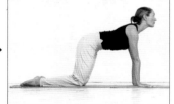 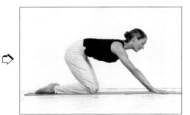

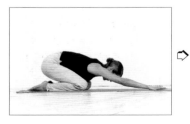 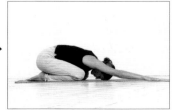 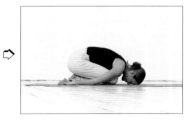

CHILD'S POSE RELAXATION

①   Focus on the base of the spine. Try and imagine each inhalation bringing fresh energy to that part of the body.

②   Now inhale the energy all the way up the spine, like the mercury rising in a thermometer. Pause when the energy has reached the top of the spine.

③   Exhale the energy slowly down the spine. Repeat the inhalation and exhalation for as long as you need for the body to completely relax.

④   Always be gentle with the breath, think of it as a fine breeze.

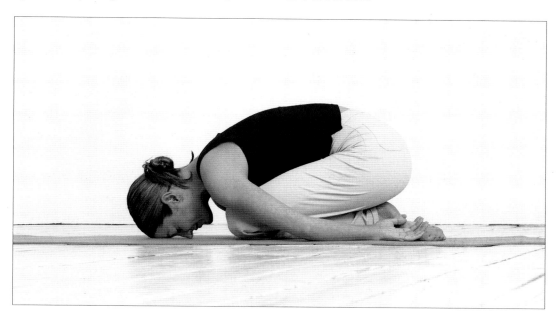

Benefits
- ✓ It calms and tones the nervous system.
- ✓ It limbers the spine, shoulders and legs.
- ✓ It stretches the neck and the back.
- ✓ The circulation is improved and the flow of blood is brought to the facial tissues and the scalp.
- ✓ The tummy is massaged relieving constipation and helping digestion.

Mistakes
- ✗ Not relaxing!!!! This is meant to be comfortable, just let go!

General Warning
- ⫶ If you have knee or hip problems you may find it uncomfortable to remain in this position for long periods of time.

The Seated Sequence

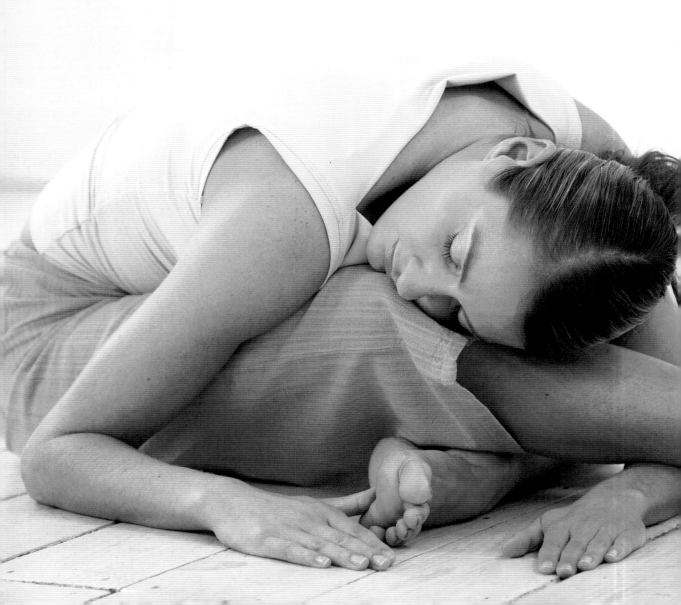

Although most of these postures are performed from a seated position a few are included here which are practised on all-fours. The initial and final relaxation may be done sitting in a chair but all the postures in this sequence should be done without a chair so please do try to get used to sitting cross-legged. Try placing the edge of a small folded cushion or pillow underneath your sit bones, the pointy bones in the middle of your buttocks. This lifts the tailbone, allows the knees and hips to soften and open and keeps the spine straight. Throughout this sequence be aware of the position of your spine. Don't slouch forward.

SEATED RELAXATION

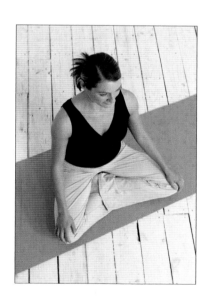

①   Sit comfortably in a cross-legged position. Have the back straight and the chest open to allow the lungs to work at the maximum efficiency. Rest your hands on your knees. If you are sitting on a chair have your legs hip-width apart.

②   Breathe comfortably and naturally. Imagine an invisible cord attached to the crown of your head pulling you straighter and straighter. Keep your awareness on the spine and keep lengthening and straightening. Lift up out of your waist, but do try to keep the entire body relaxed, especially in the hips and knees.

③   Remain here for a couple of minutes, simply observing your breathing and being aware of how your body is feeling. Try doing the full yogic breathing slowly (see page 25).

Benefits
✓ It opens the hips.
✓ The spine gets to lengthen.
✓ It facilitates mental and physical balance without any pain or strain.

Mistakes
✗ Having poor posture with the spine curved and the shoulders hunched forward.

General Warning
⁚ This posture can be very strong on the hips and knees. If you have any problems with these areas be aware of how your body feels at all times.

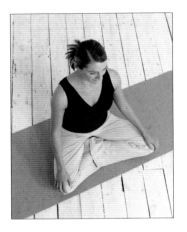

NECK RELEASE

Sit comfortably in a cross-legged position. If needed, put a cushion under the buttocks in order to lift your tailbone. Straighten the spine and look straight ahead, lengthening the back of the neck. Place the hands on the knees.

① Interlock your fingers behind your head so that your palms are flat on the head just behind each ear and your elbows are pointing out to the sides.

② Inhale. As you exhale, take your chin in towards your chest and bring the elbows together in front of your face. Concentrate on relaxing your shoulders and allowing the weight of your hands to rest on the back of the head; this will stretch the back of your neck and gently move your chin closer to your chest.

③ Inhale and open the elbows wide again and lift the chin so that it is parallel to the floor.

④ Repeat this 3 to 6 times focusing on slow steady movement and feeling the work in the shoulders and the back of the neck.

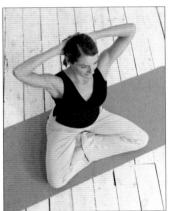

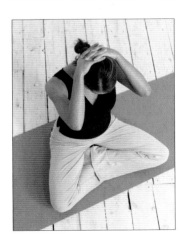

Benefits

✓ Tension from the neck is released.

✓ It stretches the neck, back and shoulder muscles.

✓ A great one to do at a desk!!!!

Mistakes

✗ The shoulders are lifted instead of relaxed.

✗ The posture goes when the neck moves downwards. Keep the back straight and lengthened throughout.

A QUICK MASSAGE

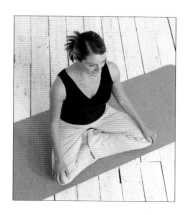

Sit comfortably in a cross-legged position as before.

①   While maintaining a steady and natural breathing rhythm, gently massage your shoulder, focusing especially on any areas of tightness. Feel the muscles warm up as you massage them.

②   Now massage down your arm and hand and fingers.

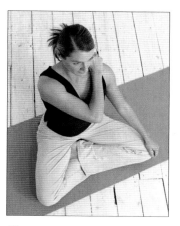

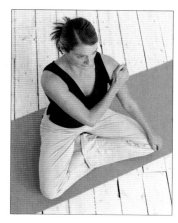

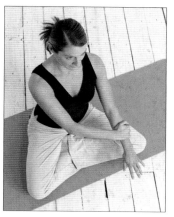

③   Don't worry too much about technique here; this is about making yourself feel a bit looser and more relaxed. Enjoy giving yourself some attention.

④   Continue massaging for about thirty seconds to a minute.

⑤   Then repeat on the other shoulder, arm and hand.

Benefits

✓   It brings the blood to the surface of the body, releases tension and feels great!

SHOULDER ROLLS

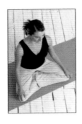

Sit comfortably in a cross-legged position as before.

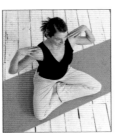

①   Place your fingers on your shoulders with your elbows pointing straight out to the side. Don't hunch your shoulders here; think of space between your shoulders and ears. Work the elbows back so that there is a straight line from one elbow, through the shoulders and along to the other elbow. Relax and breathe.

②   On an inhalation, move your elbows down so that your arms are in line with the torso, then forwards and up so that the elbows meet together in front of the face. On the exhalation take the elbows outwards, backwards and down so that they return to the starting position.

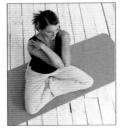

③   Imagine pencils are attached to your elbows and you are drawing huge circles as you move them around. Make the movement steady and smooth.

④   Circle in one direction 3 to 6 times and then reverse and repeat going the other way.

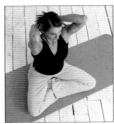

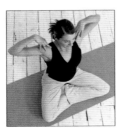

Benefits

✓ It relieves the strain of driving and office work.

✓ It maintains the shape of the shoulders and the chest.

Mistakes

✗ Loss of posture. Keep the body straight.

✗ Your head moves around. Keep it still.

✗ You don't make large enough circles with your elbows.

General Warning

❗ If you have had dislocated shoulders take great care.

A CHEST STRETCH

Sit comfortably in a cross-legged position as before.

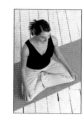

① Interlock the fingers behind the body with the arms as straight as possible. Breathe a few times in this position. You should feel the chest open and the shoulders pulled back and down. Relax here for a few moments.

② Press down through the hands as if you were trying to touch your knuckles to the floor. Keep your spine as straight as possible so that the pressure opens your chest and shoulders more. Make sure your tummy is pulled in to stop your lower back over-arching. Keep looking straight ahead and keep your chin parallel to the floor. Maintain the downward pressure for a few breaths and then relax. Repeat this 3 to 6 times.

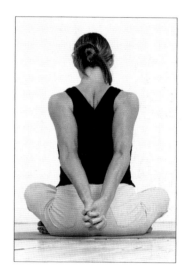

③ If this is uncomfortable, try placing your fingertips on the floor directly behind you, pointing away from the buttocks. Breathe deeply and feel the chest opening and the shoulders pulling down and back. Focus on keeping your chin parallel and your spine lengthened.

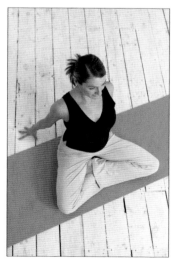

Benefits

✓ A great release for the chest muscles and the shoulder blades.

✓ A good position to help your posture if you are sitting a lot at a desk.

✓ It tones the arms and strengthens the wrists.

Mistakes

✗ Poking the chin forward, straining the neck and the back. Keep relaxed and straight.

✗ No downward pressure on the wrists and the arms are bending.

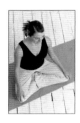

EAGLE ARMS

Sit comfortably in a cross-legged position as before.

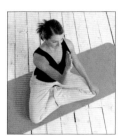

①   Take the right arm and straighten it in front of you. Now bend the arm so that the fingers are pointing up at the ceiling and the palm is facing to the left. The arm is in front of your face. The elbow should roughly be in line with the shoulder.

②   Bend the left arm underneath the right, so that the right elbow is resting pretty much on top of the left elbow crook. The left arm should be bent so that the fingers point up and the left palm is facing the opposite direction to the right palm.

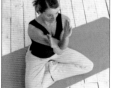

③   Try to bring the back of the hands together. If they touch, then take the shortest hand and bring it towards your face, and then sideways and back so that the fingers touch the palm of the higher hand. Try to bring the hands into a prayer position.

④   Concentrate throughout on keeping the elbows parallel to the shoulders and keeping the back straight and neck straight. Stay here and breathe. You could even close your eyes and work on slow, full breathing.

⑤   Hold for 5 to 10 long, steady breaths and then repeat on the other side.

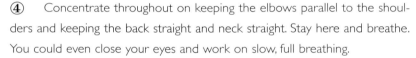

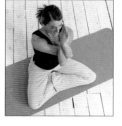

Benefits

✓ It improves circulation in the arms.

✓ It is a great release for the back and shoulders.

Mistakes

✗ Posture is lost. Keep the back straight and lengthened.

✗ An incorrect arm position.

General Warning

❗ This is a very demanding stretch for the shoulders. If you have had problems in that area be careful.

CHOPPING WOOD

Sitting on your buttocks, extend your legs out in front of you, heels pressing down and away. Soften your knees and thighs. Place the palms flat on the floor to either side of your hips and press down through your palms while straightening the spine and allowing your tailbone to continue to soften towards the floor. Relax and breathe.

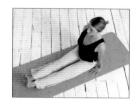

① Extend your arms in front of you, parallel to the floor, and clasp your hands.

② Exhale, and move your upper body back as far as is comfortable, if you feel any strain in the lower back you've gone too far. All the tension here should be in the stomach not the back. Feel the tail-bone pressing down through the buttocks. Keep your spine long and make sure your arms don't go above shoulder height. Keep looking forwards and think of gently releasing beneath the armpits. Pull the tummy down and in towards the spine.

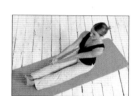

③ Inhale and see-saw your body forward, so that your hands move towards your feet. Keep the arms at the same height throughout, parallel to the floor. Press down through the buttocks and make sure you are bending from the hips and not just slouching forward and back with the upper back. It doesn't matter how far you go in each direction, it is about feeling the work in the stomach area.

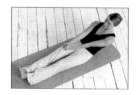

④ Repeat 8 to 16 times. Get a rhythm going. This is a great posture for warming up the body at any time.

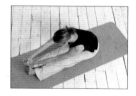

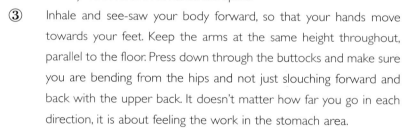

Benefits

✓ The stomach, pelvis and trunk of the body are toned.

✓ The hamstrings are stretched.

✓ The back is stretched and lengthened.

Mistakes

✗ Bad posture. Keep lifting from the hips.

✗ The arms are dropped or raised. Keep them parallel to the floor.

✗ The legs bend.

✗ The neck is strained through not using the tummy enough.

General Warning

❗ Know your own limitations on this stretch. Don't try and go too fast at first.

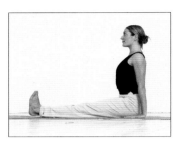

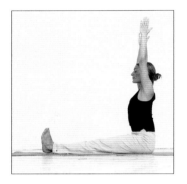

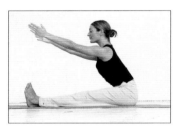

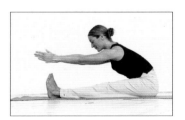

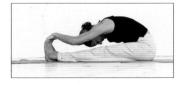

SEATED FORWARD BEND

Sitting on your buttocks, extend your legs out in front of you, heels pressing down and away. Soften your knees and thighs. Place the palms flat on the floor to either side of your hips and press down through your palms while also straightening the spine and allowing your tailbone to continue to soften towards the floor. Relax and breathe.

① Lift up through the spine and waist. Inhale and take your arms out to the side and then reach them straight up to the sky, in line with the ears and with the palms facing each other. Look up, reach up, try and touch the ceiling, and feel the muscles on both sides of your body stretching.

② Exhale and try to bend forward from the hips, not from the waist. Think of reaching up and forward with your hands, so that the chest comes forward as you bend. Keep looking in front of you, but allow the neck to stay relaxed and extended. Don't poke the chin forward.

③ As you bend forward, place your hands on the legs or the feet and hold them as you breathe. Remember to go only as far as the body allows today, and keep thinking of the back lengthening and straightening. Relax, soften the knees just a little, and stay here for as long as you can focus on the breath.

④ While holding this posture, the arms can be used to gently further the stretch. Bend the elbows back slightly. This should pull your upper body a bit closer to the legs. The aim is to rest the front of your body flat on your legs.

⑤ Use the exhalation to stretch out of the hips, lengthen the spine and feel the chest dropping.

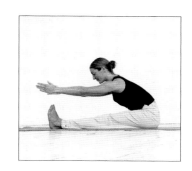

⑥ To come out of the posture, reach the arms forwards and up. Allow the upper body to follow this movement naturally and be aware of keeping the head and the neck relaxed. When the arms are straight up again, take one more stretch and then relax the arms down by the sides.

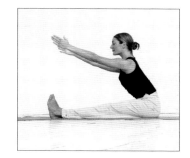

⑦ If your hamstrings are extremely stiff, you may wish to use a strap or a belt to help you. Put the strap around the soles of your feet and hold on to both ends. Tighten your grip on the strap and, as you bend forward from the hips, lengthening up through the body, keep the strap absolutely taut, with the elbows back and in, the chest open, the legs straight and looking forward. Keep lengthening as before and think of relaxing the hamstrings as you bend forward.

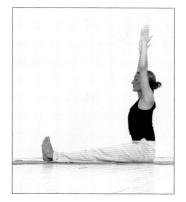

Benefits

✓ It massages the tummy and the internal organs.
✓ It tones and stimulates the digestive organs and the kidneys.
✓ It rejuvenates the spine.
✓ It regulates pancreas function, which helps people with diabetes.
✓ It strengthens and stretches the hamstrings and the spine.
✓ It relieves compression of the spine.
✓ It removes excess weight in the tummy area.
✓ It brings fresh blood to the pelvis, improving the health of the reproductive organs.

Mistakes

✗ The legs are bent.
✗ The back is rounded and the head drops. Keep coming forward with the chest.
✗ The feet roll out instead of being parallel and flexed.
✗ There is shoulder tension. Relax.

General Warning

❗ Anyone with a slipped disc, sciatica or extremely tight hamstrings should take this posture very slowly.

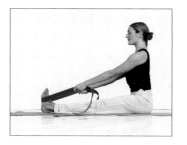

CRADLING LOTUS

Sitting on your buttocks, extend your legs out in front of you, heels pressing down and away. Soften your knees and thighs. Place the palms flat on the floor to either side of your hips and press down through your palms. Straighten the spine and allow your tailbone to continue to soften towards the floor. Relax and breathe.

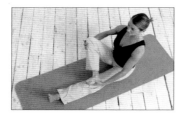 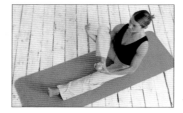 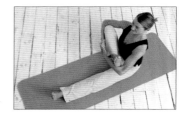

① Bend the right leg and hold the knee underneath with the right hand. Now take your left hand and hold the right foot. Try and keep the lower leg parallel to the floor. Gently rock the right leg from side to side.

② To make this more of a challenge, put your right arm underneath and through the right leg so that it supports the entire weight of the leg. Be careful of the back when you do this, it will want to collapse forward. Think of that invisible string pulling straight up through the crown of your head.

③ For even more of a challenge, wrap your left arm around the right leg also, so that the right foot is tucked into the inside of the left elbow or even resting on the upper part of the left arm. Imagine you are holding a baby. Stay here, keep rocking if you want to and breathe, keeping the body lengthened.

④ Hold the position for 5 to 10 long steady breaths and then repeat with the other leg.

Benefits
✓ The hips and buttocks are opened and stretched.
✓ The flexibility of the hips, legs and feet is improved.

Mistakes
✗ Bad posture. Always lift up through the hips and waist.
✗ Bending the opposite leg.

General Warning
❗ Anyone with hip problems or bad knees should be careful doing this one.

CAT

Come onto all fours. The hands should be directly beneath the shoulders and the knees should be directly below the hips. Feel the spine lengthen from both ends of the body in this position. Relax and breathe.

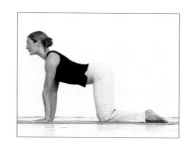

① Inhale, and look directly forward. You should feel the spine straighten and the lower back slightly relax down in a natural curve. Keep your shoulders away from the ears by working the muscles underneath the armpits. Think of the buttocks extending behind you and your chest coming forward. Continue to press down through the palms and the knees. Remember to spread out your fingers.

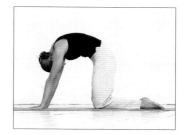

② Exhale and curl your back upward, as if your belly button is trying to touch the ceiling, and allow your head and tailbone to release down towards the floor. Look at your knees as your head sinks, but be aware of your neck as it stretches. Continue to exert pressure through the palms and knees.

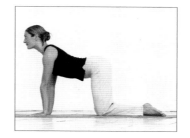

③ Inhale and come back to the starting position and repeat 6 to 12 times.

④ Focus on making the movements match your slow, steady breathing. This is a back stretch, so always be aware of how your spine is feeling.

Benefits
✓ It relieves an aching back.
✓ It strengthens the spine.
✓ It tones the arms.
✓ It reduces tummy fat.
✓ It tones the nervous system.
✓ It improves circulation.
✓ It aids digestion.
✓ It helps returns the uterus back to normal position after giving birth.

Mistakes
✗ Holding the neck stiff.
✗ Not having the shoulders directly over the hands and the hips over the feet.

General Warning
‼ If your knees are uncomfortable in this position, try putting a cushion under them. The benefits of this stretch are too good to miss just because your knees ache a little

INVERTED V

Come on to all fours. The hands should be directly beneath the shoulders and the knees should be directly below the hips. Feel the spine lengthen from both ends of the body in this position. Relax and breathe.

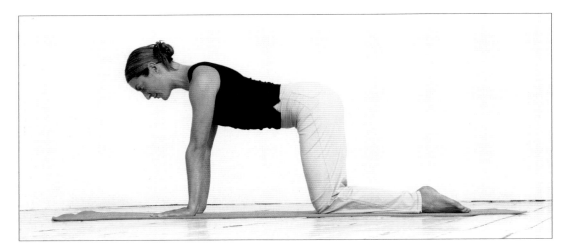

①   Inhale. On the exhalation tuck the toes under, and push the palms into the floor, keeping your fingers spread. Lift your bottom up towards the ceiling, and try to press your heels into the floor. Stay in this position and breathe.

②   You have four points of contact with the floor: both hands and both feet, push them into the floor to assist the pose. Now, imagine you have two balloons attached to you, one to your bottom and one to your hips, which pull you up straight.

③   Constantly think about stretching the hamstrings by lifting the tailbone towards the ceiling and simultaneously pressing the heels into the floor.

④   Think of the back lengthening into a straight line with the arms. You may find your palms slipping forward initially. This is probably due to your weight being distributed at too much of a diagonal, instead of going straight down. When you press down through the palms, think of weight going through the part of the palm closest to the wrist, that ridge at the bottom of your hand. That's where the weight should go through, but don't forget the fingers — they need to be spread out fully.

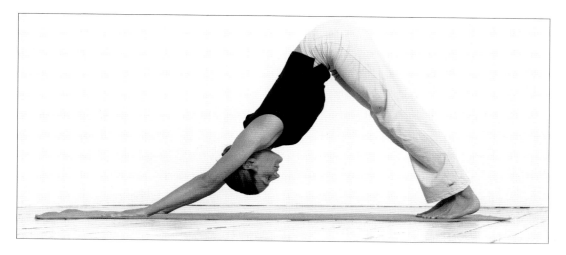

⑤ Relax the shoulders and feel them sinking, opening and stretching. Keep lifting the kneecaps and make your thighs strong.

⑥ Keep breathing and rest in Child's Pose (see page 61) when you need to. Repeat 3 to 6 times focusing on the breathing and feeling the body relax into the position.

Benefits

✓ It strengthens and tones the arms and the legs.

✓ It releases the spine and alleviates back problems.

✓ It releases tight calves and hamstrings.

✓ The circulation is stimulated in the upper spine and the shoulder blades.

Mistakes

✗ The fingers of the hands are not spread out. The palms are not pressed down into the floor.

✗ There is too much weight on the arms because the shoulders are too far forward over the hands. Let the shoulders sink, move down and back.

✗ The feet roll. Not enough thought is going into pressing the heels down into the floor.

✗ The hips are dropping instead of rising to the ceiling.

PLANK

Come on to all fours. The hands should be directly beneath the shoulders and the knees should be directly below the hips. Feel the spine lengthen from both ends of the body in this position. Relax and breathe.

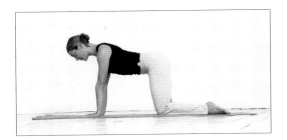
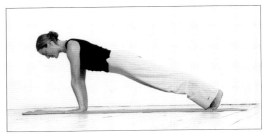

Benefits

✓ It tones the shoulders, arms, stomach, buttocks and legs.

Mistakes

✗ The spine drops out of the straight, horizontal position.

✗ You are not balanced with your hands underneath the shoulders, so too much weight is taken by the body.

✗ The neck is not in line with the spine.

General Warning

❢ If you have weak wrists, this is a great way to strengthen them, but be careful.

① Push down through the palms, spread the fingers out and move your right leg back, toes tucked under and touching the floor. Then do the same with the left leg. Make sure that your hands are still directly below the shoulders.

② Concentrate on straightening the spine. The tendency here is to allow your tummy to dip to the floor, or to raise the buttocks. Try pushing down through the heels and palms and think of lengthening the spine, this should correct you a bit.

③ Remember to pull the tummy in by exhaling and thinking of bringing the waist into the navel.

④ Hold this position for as long as comfortable. If your arms start to shake at any point, stop and relax.

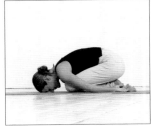

⑤ Relax into the Child's Pose (see page 61). Repeat 3 to 6 times.

HIP FLEXOR RELEASE

Come into a comfortable kneeling position. Have the knees in line with the heels. Keep the spine straight and lengthen the back of the neck. Keep the thighs pushed back and the knees soft. If your feet are uncomfortable or cramping then relax and try again shortly.

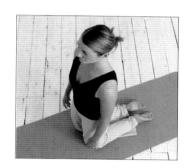

① Take your right leg forwards, foot is flat on the floor, heel directly below the knee. Place your hands on your right knee. Straighten up through the spine and neck. Press gently down through your arms to straighten up but make sure that the pressure is not going down through the knees, but rather that you are pushing back up through the body.

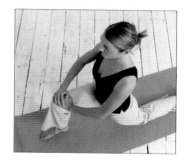

② Tighten your buttock and pelvic floor muscles and lift up out of the waist. Feel the strength being created as you push the pelvic bone forward and down, while at the same time lengthening up through your waist and lower back. Relax the shoulders, they are not doing any of the work. With each exhalation press forward and down through the hips.

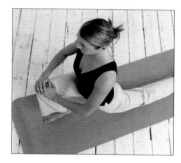

③ Hold for 3 to 6 deep breaths and then release the right leg. Feel the left hip release and the thigh lengthen. Repeat 3 to 6 times and then repeat on the left leg.

Benefits
- ✓ Great for people who spend time seated.
- ✓ It works on increasing the mobility of the hip.
- ✓ It tones the buttocks.
- ✓ It works on the stomach and calf muscles which helps increase general stability.
- ✓ It releases the thigh muscle.

Mistakes
- ✗ The knee is not directly over the foot.
- ✗ The posture is allowed to slump.
- ✗ No work is done in the stomach, and tension is allowed to come into the shoulders.

General Warning
- ❗ Take great care if you have knee problems. If this posture is uncomfortable try it with a cushion under the bent knee.

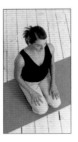

PALMING

Come into a comfortable kneeling position. Have the knees in a line with the heel. Keep the spine straight and lengthen the back of the neck. Keep the thighs pushed back and the knees soft. If your feet are uncomfortable or cramping then relax and try again shortly. Sit back on the heels, with the front of the feet flat on the floor. Relax and try to keep the weight going down through the buttocks and heels. This can be quite extreme for beginners so take your time, it's just that the front of the feet are not used to being bent like this. If kneeling isn't comfortable, you can sit on a chair.

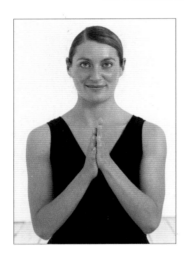

① Rub your palms together in front of you. Really move them quickly and start to generate some heat.

② When your hands feel quite warm, if not hot, then cup your palms over your closed eyes and hold them there.

③ Relax your shoulders and breathe slowly.

④ Repeat 1 to 3 times.

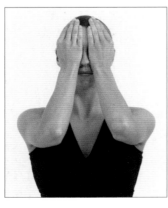

Benefits

✓ It brings energy and sparkle to the eyes.

✓ It stimulates the circulation of the liquid that runs between the cornea and lens of the eye.

Mistakes

✗ The hands are not cupped.

✗ The fingers are spread.

✗ The shoulders are tense.

LION

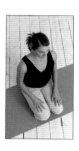

Come into a comfortable kneeling position with the buttocks resting on the heels. Keep the back straight and neck lengthened and think of a weight going straight down your spine, through the buttocks and heels and down into the floor. If kneeling isn't comfortable, you can sit on a chair.

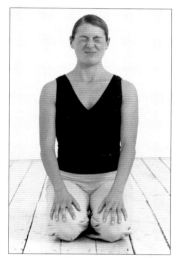

①   Place your hands on your knees and straighten the body.

②   Inhale and squeeze your face together, imagine you have just tasted something bitter.

③   Now, do this all at once: as you exhale through your mouth, stick your tongue out (try and touch your chin with your tongue), look up with wide eyes, your body should come slightly forward, the hands should flex, and all that air should pour out in a long pant. No baby lions!!! Rahhhhhhhhhhh.

④   Repeat 3 to 6 times.

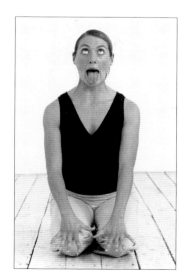

Benefits

✓ Releases feelings of aggression.

✓ It tones the face and the neck. It's a mini facelift!

✓ It relieves sore throats.

✓ It cleans the tongue and fights bad breath.

✓ It helps with speech, and can help to cure a stammer if practised.

Mistakes

✗ You don't exhale for long enough. Make it slow and steady.

✗ The hands don't flex.

✗ The eyes don't look up.

✗ You're a baby lion – let's hear you!!

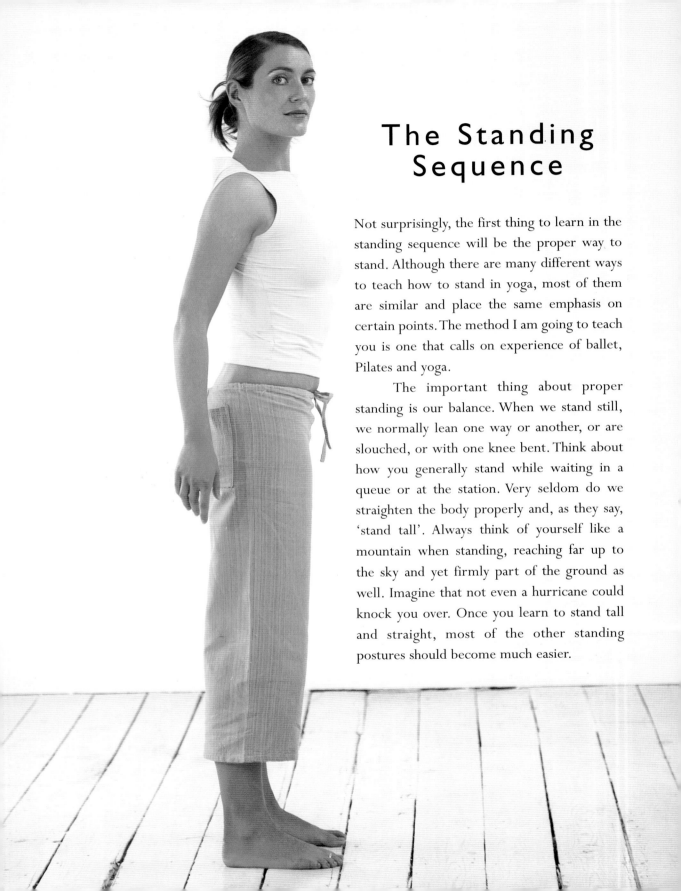

The Standing Sequence

Not surprisingly, the first thing to learn in the standing sequence will be the proper way to stand. Although there are many different ways to teach how to stand in yoga, most of them are similar and place the same emphasis on certain points. The method I am going to teach you is one that calls on experience of ballet, Pilates and yoga.

The important thing about proper standing is our balance. When we stand still, we normally lean one way or another, or are slouched, or with one knee bent. Think about how you generally stand while waiting in a queue or at the station. Very seldom do we straighten the body properly and, as they say, 'stand tall'. Always think of yourself like a mountain when standing, reaching far up to the sky and yet firmly part of the ground as well. Imagine that not even a hurricane could knock you over. Once you learn to stand tall and straight, most of the other standing postures should become much easier.

STANDING POSTURE

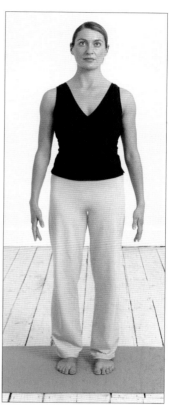

①   Stand with your legs hip-width apart. Remember that a hip's width is taken from just inside the hip bone and not from the outer edges of your legs. There is a big difference!! The outside of your feet should be parallel, so that the insides of your feet seem to be coming closer together at the toes.

②   Soften the knees and push the thighs back very slightly, so you can just feel the legs straighten and the buttocks firm a little.

③   Relax the arms down by your sides and have the fingers relaxed and pointed down, palms facing the body. Soften the shoulders down and back so the arms are down by the sides of the body not in front.

④   Feel the floor. Spread your toes (without the heels moving) and have the weight going through the centre of your feet. This means your weight is evenly distributed between the front and the back of the foot.

⑤   Lift up out of the waist. Allow your spine to extend all the way up, as that invisible string attached to the crown of your head pulls you higher and higher. Don't lift the shoulders. Feel the body descending from the waist down and ascending from the waist up.

⑥   Breathe comfortably and slowly. Remain in this posture until you feel tall, balanced, and strong.

Benefits

✓ It concentrates on the correct alignment of the spine and on good posture.

✓ It brings about lightness of mind and body through correct alignment.

✓ This is great for correcting generally poor posture!!

Mistakes

✗ Too much weight on the heels or toes changes the whole alignment of the body. Keep the weight evenly distributed.

✗ The tummy sags, keep it tucked in.

✗ The shoulders are hunched. Relax.

✗ The chin juts forward. Lengthen the back of the neck and allow your chin to drop slightly towards the chest so that you are looking straight ahead.

TABLE TOP

Stand facing a wall and about an arm's length away from it. Bend forward with one arm stretched forward and one back. If you can't touch the wall, you are too far away, but if you touch it before the hamstrings have stretched, you are too close. The correct distance is where you are able to touch the wall just as you feel the hamstrings begin to stretch. Adjust your feet in this position so they are parallel and hip-width apart, with the legs directly under the hips.

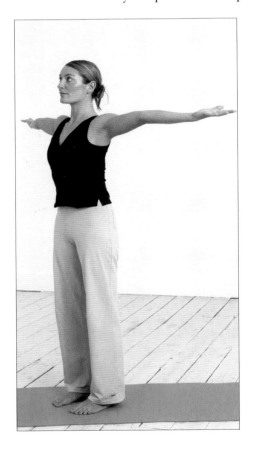

①   Extend the arms straight out and up and stretch the entire spine. Look up and stretch. I like to do this action with the palms facing each other, it gives me more extension and a feeling of space. I can really pull up from my fingertips. Lift up out of the hips, spine elongating.

②   Exhale and bend through the hips, keeping the back straight by reaching forwards and up as you go down. Take the hands, arms and upper body forward until you reach the wall. You are aiming to be flat, like a table top, so that the body is at a 90° angle to the hips. Press the palms into the wall.

③   The head is in line with the arms. Think of extending the crown of your head forwards and extending your spine from the first to the last vertebra.

④   Try and keep the legs straight, kneecaps lifted, weight going evenly down through the feet and up into the hips.

⑤   Breathe here. Gently push the bottom back towards the opposite wall to stretch the spine and

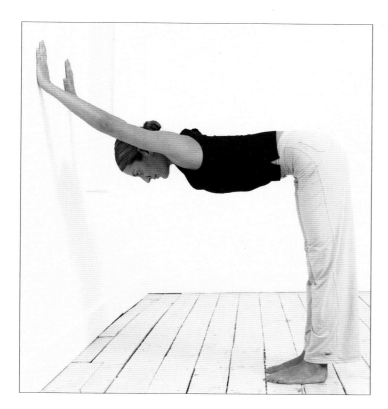

Benefits

✔ It increases the flexibility of the hip joints and the hamstrings.

✔ It opens the shoulders and the chest and increases mobility in the shoulder socket.

✔ It rejuvenates the spine.

✔ It strengthens the feet, ankles and thighs.

Mistakes

✗ Incorrect alignment of the hips to the legs. The hips should be at 90° and directly above the feet. Your legs should be straight.

✗ The spine doesn't lengthen, and the hips don't push backwards. Stick that bum out!

✗ The knees bend.

✗ Bending from the waist not the hips.

✗ The feet are too far apart.

✗ Too much weight on the arms. The weight should be back and down through the hips and legs.

hamstrings. Keep the hands where they are, feeling the spine trying to lengthen. Relax the shoulders and feel them sink towards the floor. You will feel this stretch in the backs of the legs.

⑥ Hold this posture for 5 to 10 long, steady breaths, then inhale and reach forward and up with the arms, drop the tailbone down and lift up through the hips. When the arms are back above the head, relax and drop them to your sides.

⑦ Repeat 3, 6, 9 or 12 times.

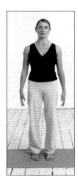

STANDING FORWARD BEND AND ROLL UP

Stand correctly as described in the Standing Posture on page 81.

①   Inhale and take the arms slowly out to the sides and then above the head. Reach up, look up and feel the entire body lengthen.

②   Exhale and bend from the hips, reaching forward and up with your arms as you bend. Think of your bottom sticking out as you reach forwards with the arms and the body. Think of the spine constantly lengthening as you move downwards. The weight should be even on the feet and pushing straight down.

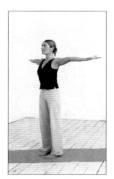 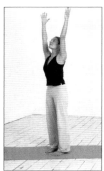 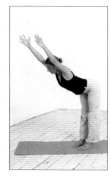 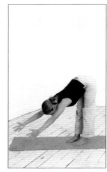 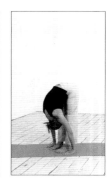

③   When you have reached as far as you can go, relax the head and arms and allow them to dangle freely. If your hands reach the floor, try and flatten the palms by lengthening the spine on an inhalation and allowing the body to bend further at the hips on an exhalation. Focus on keeping the back lengthened throughout.

④   You will feel this stretch in the backs of the legs. Keep relaxing any areas of discomfort and breathing through the stretch. You will know if you have gone too far. Just allow the body to go as far as it wants to, but make sure you get a good stretch.

⑤   Hold for up to 10 slow, steady breaths and then soften the knees slightly, inhale and curl up, vertebra by vertebra, keeping your hands and head heavy until the entire spine has straightened itself out. Only then should the shoulders drop back and the neck straighten.

⑥   Repeat 3 to 6 times.

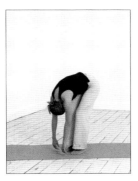 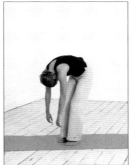 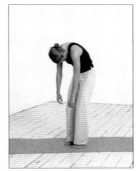 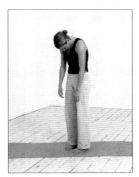

Benefits
✓ It is great for any tummy problems.
✓ It tones the tummy, removing excess weight.
✓ It improves digestion and helps relieve constipation.
✓ It tones the spinal nerves.
✓ It makes the spine supple.

Mistakes
✗ Bending from the waist not from the hips.
✗ Having the shoulders slouched forward and not relaxed.
✗ Having the knees bent. Keep the legs straight.
✗ Having the weight forward or back, keep it balanced and even.

General Warning
⁝ If you have had a prolapsed disc then this posture should be done with caution.

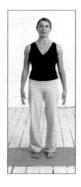

WARRIOR 1

Stand correctly as described in the Standing Posture on page 81.

① Step or jump so that the legs are just over a metre apart. The feet should be parallel and the back straight.

② Turn your right foot around 90° so that it is pointing out to the side. Press down through your left heel.

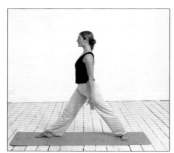

③ Turn the body and hips to face your right leg. Your left foot may have to turn inward to help you balance the pose. Keep your weight going through your left heel. Your hips should be facing your right foot.

④ Bend your right leg so that your knee is eventually directly over the toes of your right foot. Your left leg will want to bend, keep it straight. Feel the leg working right down into the outside of that left foot. You don't want your foot to roll inwards. Lift up through the upper body, especially through the waist.

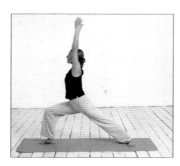

⑤ Take your arms straight up so your fingers are pointing to the ceiling, palms facing each other. Keep your shoulders down, they will want to wander up round the ears.

⑥ Breathe in this position for up to 6 deep breaths or for however long you are comfortable. Keep straightening and pushing down through the left leg and foot.

⑦ Repeat on the other side.

Benefits Common to Warrior 1 and 2
✓ They tone the legs, bum, arms and stomach.
✓ They relieve stiffness in the hips and the legs.
✓ They strengthen the legs.
✓ They improve balance and concentration.
✓ They relieve cramp in the thighs and calves.

Mistakes Common in Warrior 1 and 2
✗ Both legs are bent and the knee twists out.
✗ The hip alignment is incorrect.
✗ You have floppy arms.

WARRIOR 2

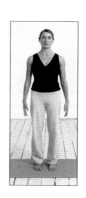

Stand correctly as described in the Standing Posture on page 81.

①   Step or jump so that your legs are just over a metre apart. The feet should be parallel and the back straight. The hips should face forward and should remain there throughout.

②   Turn your right foot around 90° so that it is pointing out to the side. Now press down through the left heel. Keep the hips straight.

③   Bring your arms up to shoulder height, with the palms facing down. Turn your head to look along your right arm towards your right hand.

④   Pressing through your left heel, bend your right leg but keep the body straight up and the arms extended. The right leg should be bent so that your knee is directly over your toes. Make sure the back leg is straight and powerful. Keep working it and keep pressing the left heel down.

⑤   Hold for up to 6 long, deep breaths and then release the pressure on your left leg and straighten the right leg. Drop the arms and look forward.

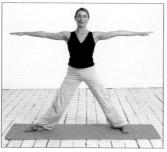
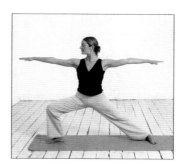

⑥   Repeat on the left side.

✗   The weight is not evenly distributed between the feet. Keep that balance.

✗   The bent knee is not over the toes.

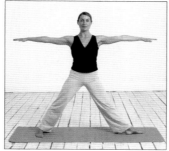
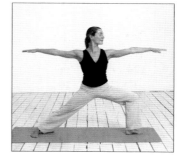

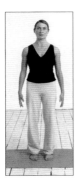

TREE

Stand correctly as described in the Standing Posture on page 81.

    This is a balancing posture so it might be good to be near a wall at first until your confidence builds up. Whenever you are in a balancing posture try to find a point of focus somewhere and stay concentrated on that point. Ideally, it should be at eye height so that your head remains balanced.

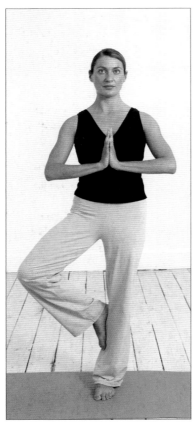

①   Have your feet hip-width apart. Place your right foot on your left calf. If it is comfortable here then try to bring the foot higher up the leg, although it should never be resting against your knee. Avoid putting direct pressure on the knee at all times! Make sure the supporting leg remains straight and keep the weight driving down through the foot.

②   Try and keep the hips square to the front of the room. Take your hands into a prayer position and breathe in this posture. Keep your focus and think about your balance.

③   Lift up out of the hips and waist, lengthen the back and at the same time send your weight down through the supporting leg, grounding you. It's really important to keep lifting up out of the waist and the upper body as this will help you have good posture. Visualize a tree growing, it's like your body lifting and lengthening but at the same time your feet are grounding you, like the roots.

④   If you would like to try a more advanced version, take your arms up above the head, keeping your shoulders relaxed. Bring the palms together at the top and straighten the arms, trying to relax the shoulders so that the arms are touching the ears. Extend upwards and keep sending weight down through the supporting leg.

⑤ Always keep your eyes focused on a particular point, but if you want to try a bit of fun then close your eyes and see what it does to your balance. And remember to keep your tummy in!

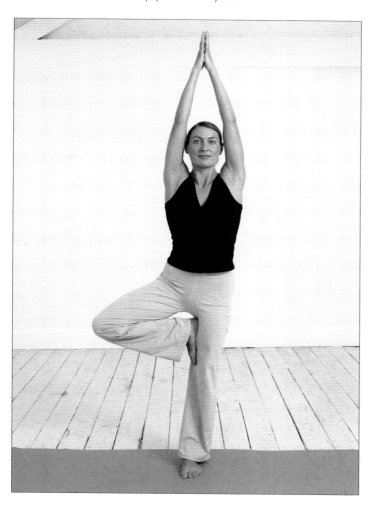

Benefits

✓ It tones the legs, bum, tummy and ankles.
✓ It improves balance and poise.
✓ It improves concentration.
✓ It tones the arms.
✓ It works on posture.

Mistakes

✗ You have the body leaning to one side or the hips twisting.
✗ The supporting knee is bent.
✗ The palms are not flat together.
✗ The elbows are bent. Keep the arms straight.
✗ The eyes are looking down.
✗ The mind is lacking proper concentration.

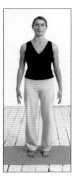

MINI TRIANGLE

Stand correctly as described in the Standing Posture on page 81.

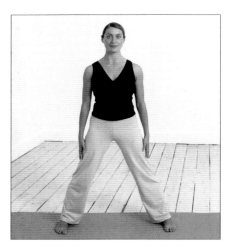

① Step or jump so that your legs are about a metre apart. Make sure the outsides of the feet are parallel with each other.

② Rest your right hand on the outside of the right thigh.

③ Inhale. Take your left arm sideways and up so it is alongside the left ear, pointing straight up and with the palm facing in. Lift straight up through the left arm, feeling the spine lengthen.

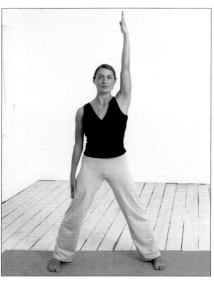

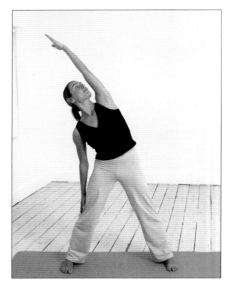

④ Exhale and reach your palm over to the right, bending sideways from the hips and sliding the right hand down the right leg as you bend. Go as far as you can.

⑤ Hold the posture and breathe, keeping your tummy tucked in. Keep the body facing forwards, with the head looking up into the upper arm.

⑥ There is a tendency to allow the hips to twist; think of having headlights on the hipbones which must stay pointing directly forward at all times. Think of opening the left shoulder up and back so that the body stays flat at the front.

⑦ Hold for up to 10 steady breathes. Inhale and lift the arm up and back to the left. You may also push gently down through the right hand to straighten the body again.

⑧ Repeat on the left side.

⑨ Repeat 3 times.

Benefits

✓ It tones the legs.
✓ It removes stiffness in the legs and the hips.
✓ It corrects minor deformities in the legs.
✓ It relieves backaches and neck strain.
✓ It strengthens the ankles.
✓ It develops the chest and tones the arms.
✓ It pulls in the waist and aids digestion.
✓ It tones the nervous system, and alleviates nervous depression.
✓ It gives a lateral (sideways) bend of the spine and helps maintain the health of the spine by enabling it to bend in all directions.

Mistakes

✗ One or both knees are bent.
✗ The body and hips are twisted.
✗ The upper elbow is bent.
✗ The weight doesn't go down through the back of the heel.
✗ The head drops forward.
✗ The weight is not evenly distributed.
✗ The eyes look down.
✗ Too much weight is placed on the thigh.

THE FULL PROGRAMME

These postures you have been learning can also be linked together with the breath, making short or long sequences depending on how long you stay in each pose. Try to coordinate the breath with your movements. Remember, your exhalations are to help release tension and toxins out of the body, and your inhalations are a receiving of oxygen and energy. If you focus on the breath this links your body to your mind, creating your yoga.

    To give yourself a full yoga class, move fluidly through the postures in the order shown, starting with the lying sequence, then seated and standing sequences.

Lying Sequence

Corpse Pose p. 45
Big Stretch p. 46
The Ball p. 47
The Frog p. 48
Ankle Circles p. 49
Double Knee Spinal Twist p. 50
Hamstring Stretches p. 52
Double Leg Stretch p. 54
Single Leg Spinal Twist p. 55
The Bridge p. 56
Preparation for
and Full Cobra p. 58
Extended Cat and
Moving from Cobra to Child's
Pose p. 60
Child's Pose Relaxation p. 61

Seated Sequence

Sit Cross Legged p. 63
Neck Release p. 64
Quick Massage p. 65
Shoulder Rolls p. 66
Chest Stretch p. 67
Eagle Arms p. 68
Chopping Wood p. 69
Seated Forward Bend p. 70
Cradling Lotus p. 72
Cat p. 73
Inverted V p. 74
Plank p.76
Hip Flexor Release p. 77
Palming p. 78
Lion Pose p. 79

Standing Sequence

Standing Posture p. 81
Table Top p. 82
Standing Forward Bend
and Roll Up p. 84
Warrior 1 p. 86
Warrior 2 p. 87
Tree p. 88
Mini Triangle p. 90

Now, to complete the class, go on to Sun Salutation (p.103) and final relaxation (p.39).

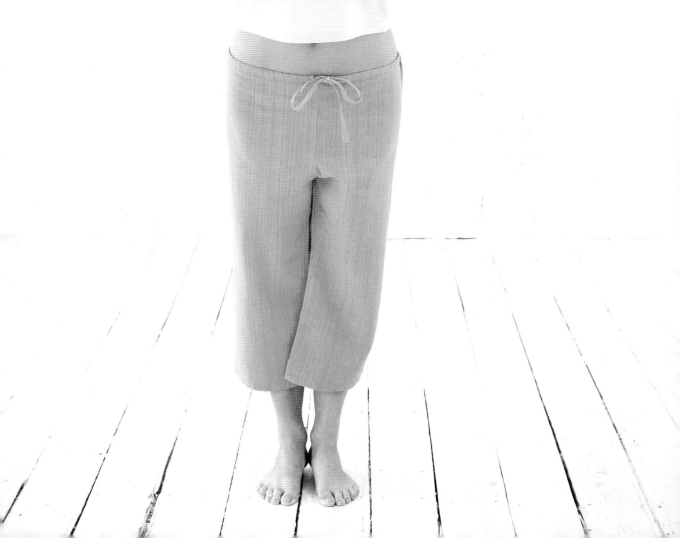

The Sun Salutation

The Sun Salutation is a great way to begin or end any day. In fact, it can be done at any time (except after eating) and it stretches just about any part of the body you want. The name in Sanskrit is surya namaskar (su-ria namas-car) and it has been a part of yoga for thousands of years. A long time ago the sun was worshipped as a god, because it brought light and heat. People must have thought that the Sun Salutation was very special because it was named after the most powerful thing in their world. It *is* special, and even if it's the only exercise you do, it can bring huge benefits.

The Sun Salutation consists of a sequence of movements that should be done in time with the breathing. For every inhalation there is an up or forward movement, and for every exhalation there is a down or backward movement. Initially, you should not worry too much about the breathing pattern. I will teach you the correct breathing, but for now, while you are learning this sequence, just begin by thinking about keeping a steady breath going. Concentrate on getting each movement correct, especially moving from one posture to another. This is the part that often causes problems for beginners. None of the postures by themselves are very difficult, but when you are expected to put them all together it can be tough at first. Take your time, and get comfortable in each posture. Sometimes it is a great help to break down the postures into threes, so that the movements between each posture are properly understood. In time, the breathing will flow naturally with the movement.

It is important that you don't go too quickly. Think about letting your body move at a steady pace throughout, so that the same amount of time is spent in each posture. Always think about relaxing any part of the body that may be tight and as you go along be aware of how different muscles are stretching. The correct speed for you is probably the speed of a good deep breath. Since each posture is done on an alternating inhalation or exhalation (except one, but more on that later) then you shouldn't be moving more quickly than your breathing!

As you become more comfortable with the movements, you should start to think about the three basic elements of the Sun Salutation: the physical postures, the breathing process and the mental attitude.

THE PHYSICAL POSTURES

There are twelve postures in the Sun Salutation. Twelve is the number of the zodiac and the number of months in a year. Understand the way that the postures join together and turn into one continuous movement. Try and flow through the sequence without thinking of each posture as an individual thing. It is all part of the entire movement.

THE BREATHING PROCESS

Work towards breathing in perfect rhythm with the movements of the body. Bring the breathing in tune with the body. As the breathing relaxes the body, the movements will become easier and your enjoyment will increase. Take proper deep inhalations and be sure to exhale fully each time, but with no strain.

THE MENTAL ATTITUDE

Be focused and aware of how both the body and the breathing are functioning. Keep the thoughts directed towards what you are doing right now, and be aware of every change as it occurs. As this awareness grows, you will suddenly discover that your breathing, body and mind are working together, in unison.

BENEFITS

The Sun Salutation has many benefits: it is said to exercise 140 different muscles; in the morning it wakes you up, stretches you, opens up your breathing, and makes you feel great! Do it whenever you want, but it is best if it is part of your daily routine, done after initial relaxation but before any other posture. Begin by trying to understand each posture and how they link together. Once you've done that try three complete rounds (one round is actually twenty-four postures, as each set of twelve is done either on the right or left side) until the breathing is comfortable and you can feel how each posture is stretching the body. After that there is no limit to how many rounds you can do. I would recommend doing no more than six complete rounds each time, but if you were doing no other postures there is no reason why you shouldn't do more.

SUN SALUTATION TECHNIQUE

The Sun Salutation begins and ends in a comfortable standing position. Before commencing, quickly check that your body is feeling fine. Take a moment to look at your breathing and make sure it is relaxed and steady. There are twelve steps to this exercise and for each step I will tell you whether the movement is accompanied by an in breath or an out breath. Don't worry too much about that at the beginning, concentrate on the movement and the technique.

ONE

a Stand straight with the feet together. Check that the weight is evenly distributed between the soles and the balls of the feet. Think of three points on the base of the foot; one underneath your heel and the other two underneath your big and little toe; your weight should be in the centre of this imaginary triangle.

b Lift up through the waist. Imagine the invisible string attached to the crown of your head pulling your entire upper body up, straightening and lengthening as it goes. Feel everything below the waist descending and everything above the waist ascending.

c Inhale and take the arms sideways, then stretch them out and up.

d Exhale and bring the arms down and into a prayer position, with the palms together level with the middle of your chest.

e Maintain the lift through your waist, feeling the tummy lift as well.

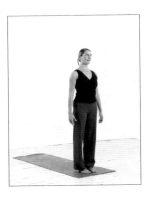 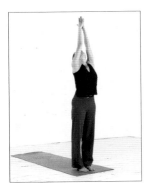 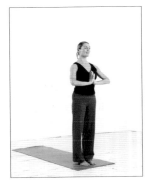

TWO

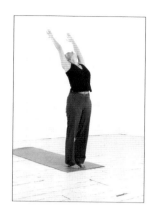

a　Inhale and take the arms straight up in front of the face, with the palms facing. The arms are reaching for the ceiling. Feel the spine stretch and lengthen.

b　Tilt the pubic bone forward and up slightly. You should feel the muscles in your bum start to work, protecting the lower back.

c　Begin to move backwards from the hips. Keep reaching up with the hands throughout. Bend backwards as far as is comfortable. If your breathing becomes restricted in any way, then you have gone too far. Don't tip the head back too much, try and keep the neck in line with the arms.

THREE

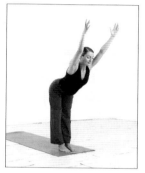

a　Exhale and bend forward from the hips, tilting your pubic bone back the other way and reaching up and forward with your arms and hands.

b　Reach towards the wall in front of you as you bend down. Imagine going through the Table Top pose, with the arms outstretched and the armpits long. Keep the back lengthened and the knees lifted into the thighs. Have your weight spread evenly through your feet, not just on the heels. Continue to fold over and try to place your hands down by your feet, with the tops of the fingers and toes in line (twenty digits in a line) and the palms pressed into the floor on either side of the feet. The body should be folded down in front of the legs. If you are able to place your hands flat then you should keep them in this exact spot throughout the next few postures until you are told to lift them again later in position Ten.

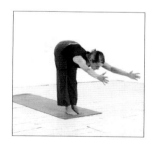

c　If your hands don't reach the floor, bend the knees to assist you. If you do this, remember to keep pressing up through the tailbone in order to stretch the hamstring muscles.

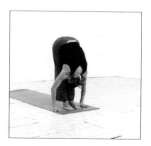

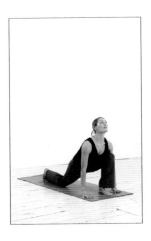

FOUR

a   Inhale deeply and press down through the hands and lift the right foot. Take a large step back with the right leg. Go as far as you can reach. Have the toes of the right foot on the floor.

b   Bend your left leg as you take the right leg back so that your left leg ends up with your left knee directly over the left toes.

c   Bring your head up and look straight ahead. Press your shoulders down and back, feeling your chest open.

d   The palms of your hands should still be flat on the floor.

e   Sink down through the pelvis, feeling the stretch in the buttocks, thighs and hamstrings.

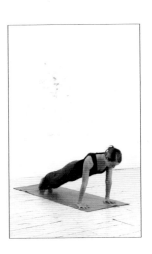

FIVE

a   Hold the breath for this movement. This is the one time a movement will be made without an inhalation or exhalation.

b   Press down through the palms. Lift the left foot and take the left leg back to meet the right. You should now be in the familiar Plank pose (see page 76).

c   The hands and arms should be directly under the shoulders, head and neck in line with the spine. You should be looking down at the floor just in front of you.

d   Don't relax the tummy, keep it strong.

e   Press the heels back and down into the floor in order to straighten the body, don't move the upper body, this is only felt in the legs.

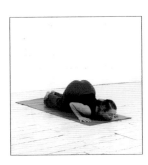

SIX

a   Before exhaling, perform the following three releases:

b   Bring your knees down to the floor.

c   Turn your toes back so that the tops of your feet are flat on the floor.

d   Push your hips and buttocks slightly backwards. Your hands should still be under your shoulders and your knees under your hips.

e   Exhale and bring the chest between the hands and the chin forward and down towards the floor. Push back through the hips and the bum while you release the downward pressure through the palms so that your bum seems to rise in the air as your chest falls between your hands. Try and make sure to keep your hands in the same position throughout.

f   Check that your elbows are tucked into the body and the shoulders are relaxed.

SEVEN

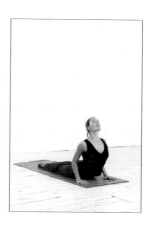

a   Inhale and slide the upper body forward and between the hands. Tucking the bum down into the floor, press forward and up with the chest so that the head lifts from the floor. Reach your head towards the far wall and ceiling. This is the Cobra pose (see page 58).

b   Keep the hands where they are and when you are unable to lift the body any more then press down through the palms to lift more. Your tummy should just remain in contact with the floor.

c   Keep your shoulders down and back, and remember to keep your elbows tucked in.

EIGHT

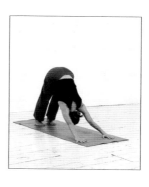

a   Exhale and tuck the toes underneath, press down through the palms to straighten the arms, push the tailbone back and up, and lift the bottom up to the ceiling into the Inverted V (see page 74).

b   Try and make the movements from Cobra into Inverted V smooth and steady. This is one to practise just by itself.

c   Use the strength of your tummy muscles, holding them in as you press down through the palms.

d   Try and keep your shoulders down and relaxed.

e   The movement should be similar to a see-saw action. Just remember: the heels are down, the legs are straight, you have strong arms, and balloons are attached to your buttocks!

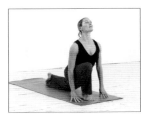

NINE

a   Inhale and bring the weight forward through the arms and lift the right foot, then step with the right foot between the hands. The left knee should drop to the floor as you step. It's really important that the foot goes between your hands for the alignment of the sequence.

b   If you find this step too much at present then take the leg as far forward as possible and help it along by taking hold of the ankle and lifting it further forward. Eventually it should be far enough forward so that the toes of the right foot and the fingers of the right hand are in line. This movement will loosen up in time, just keep practising.

c   The head should also now come up and you should feel a sinking down through your buttocks.

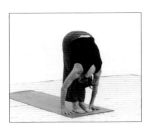

TEN

a   Exhale and press down through the right foot, push gently forward through the left foot and come back to standing, with the body folded as far down over the legs as possible.

b   The fingers and toes should all be in line on the floor with the palms pressing down. If you need to, bend your knees to get the palms flat.

ELEVEN

a   Inhale and reach forwards and up with the hands, with straight legs.

b   Allow your arms to lead the rest of your body up. Keep the neck extended and keep the back lengthened.

c   Go back through the Table Top (see page 82) as you rise all the way up to standing upright.

d   If comfortable, tilt the pubic bone forwards and up and rock back slightly as for step Two.

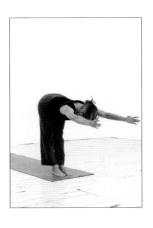

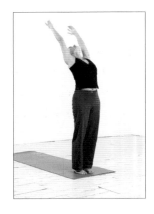

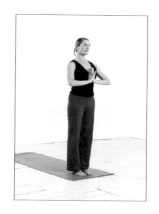

TWELVE

a   Exhale and return to the prayer position with the palms together in front of the chest.

Now you should begin again using the other leg. So now the left leg will go back first, followed by the right. And the left leg will come forwards first, followed by the right. When you have completed both sides, twenty-four steps in all, then you have done one round of the Sun Salutation.

Begin by doing a few rounds and gradually build up to 6 or 9 at a time, possibly adding one round a week.

Make sure you remember first what movement comes next. Only after having the sequence firmly in your memory should you start to add the breath to the movements.

BREATHING TIPS FOR THE SUN SALUTATION

Once you have mastered the postures and how they flow from one to another you will need to add the breath into the sequence to allow it to flow properly and get the full benefit of the postures.

Often when I'm teaching this to new students the breath gets lost, so here are a few tips to help you out and to tell you exactly when and where to breathe.

Let's start at the beginning of the sequence. Begin each movement first and then take the breath mid-way and remember to breathe deeply; the longer you breathe, the more time you have for the posture!

1   Start with the arms going out to the side and, as they meet at shoulder height, inhale, keep going with the arms and then exhale into the prayer position.

2   Stretch up with the arms and as the hands go pass the face, inhale.

3   As you bend forwards and get in the Table Top position, exhale, continuing head to knees.

4   Step the leg back and as the knee connects to the floor and the head comes up, inhale.

5   Now hold the breath and go swiftly into the Plank, do the three releases until you . . .

6   Exhale, with the chest between the hands. The body moves forward.

7   Coming up into Cobra, inhale.

8   Move into the Inverted V and, as your heels lower in this position, exhale.

9   Move your leg forward, help it along if you need to. When your knee connects to the floor and the head lifts, inhale deeply.

10   Come to standing before exhaling.

11   Move your arms forwards and when they get half way, inhale, continue the movement.

12   Exhale in the prayer position.

THE SUN SALUTATION

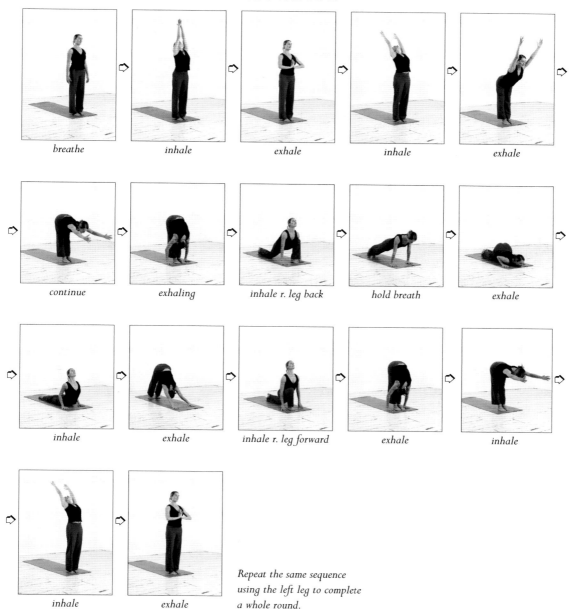

breathe

inhale

exhale

inhale

exhale

continue

exhaling

inhale r. leg back

hold breath

exhale

inhale

exhale

inhale r. leg forward

exhale

inhale

inhale

exhale

Repeat the same sequence
using the left leg to complete
a whole round.

Final Thought

Did you remember to relax at the end of your yoga practice? This is a really big part of yoga. Go back to the Final Relaxation section on page 38. Take the time to calm your body and mind after the exercise. You will feel the body relax and soften. Only then will the full benefits of your yoga be properly absorbed by your body. After that you will be ready to face anything!!

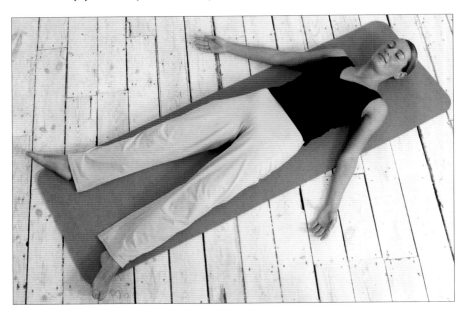

PROGRAMMES FOR LIFE – DIPPING INTO THE YOGA TOOL BOX

Daily Mini Plans

Each of these mini plans are simple ways that you can use the yoga tool box to concentrate on strengthening or relaxing certain parts of the body. Each of the plans has been designed to be done in about 15 minutes. But feel free to create your own plan. Remember to start each one with breathing and end with relaxation.

DAILY MIND TRAINING

Each day, find the same time to sit without disturbance and watch your breathing for 10 minutes. If your mind needs more to focus on then perhaps use one of the other techniques discussed in the Mind Training section on page 28.

I have indicated where you should inhale and exhale. Elsewhere just focus on breathing in rhythm with the body.

SOLUTIONS FOR SITTING FOR LONG PERIODS

This plan is aimed at those of you who do jobs involving sitting at a desk for long periods each day. For many people working in such jobs, the main problem is that the spine and neck become compressed throughout the day, the shoulders hunch forward closing the chest and the legs simply don't get a lot of activity. The combination of postures below is designed to counter each of these symptoms and to leave you feeling a little bit straighter and taller.

THE CORPSE POSE   BIG STRETCH   THE BALL

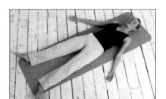
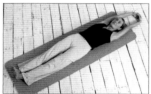
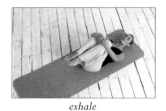

inhale   *exhale*

DOUBLE KNEE TWIST

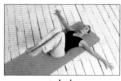
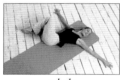
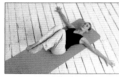
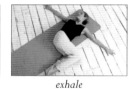

inhale   *exhale*   *inhale*   *exhale*

NECK RELEASE

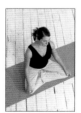
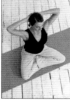
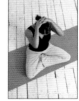

inhale   *exhale*

SHOULDER ROLLS

inhale   *inhale*   *exhale*

A CHEST STRETCH

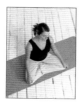 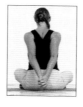 *or*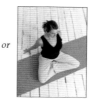

THE CAT

 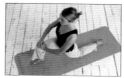 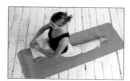

inhale   *exhale*   *inhale*

HIP FLEXOR RELEASE

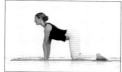 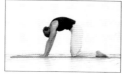 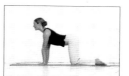

repeat on left leg

TABLE TOP

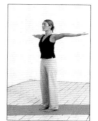

inhale   *exhale*

STIFF LEGS AND HIPS

So many of us lack flexibility around the hips and the hamstrings. This can be overcome, but you must be very patient and disciplined. Whenever you are trying to stretch out the hips and hamstrings always focus on allowing gravity to do the hard work, and just concentrate on your breathing. Make special use of the breath, always sinking into the posture further on your exhalation.

THE CORPSE POSE

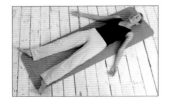

THE FROG

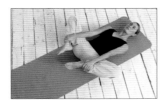

ANKLE CIRCLES

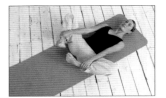

HAMSTRING STRETCHES

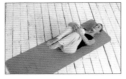
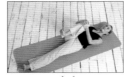
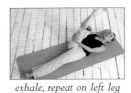

inhale   *exhale, repeat on left leg*

SEATED FORWARD BEND

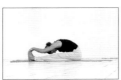

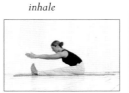

inhale   *exhale*

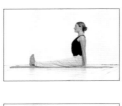
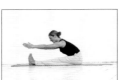

inhale to top   *exhale arms down*

CRADLING LOTUS

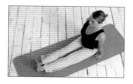 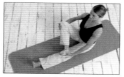 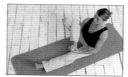 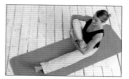

repeat on left leg

THE CAT

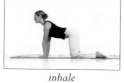 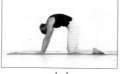 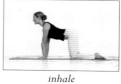

inhale   *exhale*   *inhale*

INVERTED V

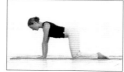 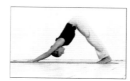

inhale   *exhale*

HIP FLEXOR RELEASE

 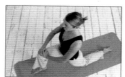 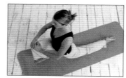

repeat on left leg

TABLE TOP

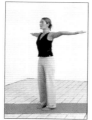 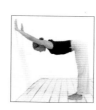

inhale   *exhale*

STANDING FORWARD BEND WITH ROLL UP

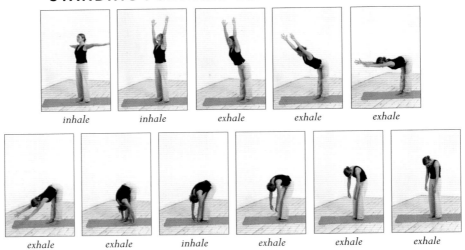

inhale   inhale   exhale   exhale   exhale

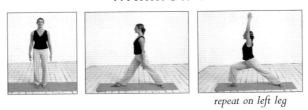

exhale   exhale   inhale   exhale   exhale   exhale

WARRIOR I

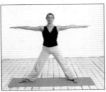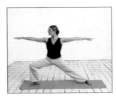

repeat on left leg

WARRIOR 2

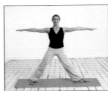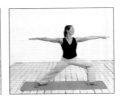

STRENGTHENING THE BACK

No part of our body is under more stress every day than our spine. It is vital that proper attention is paid to stretching and strengthening the spine continually, and all the muscles that surround it. The sequence below warms you up, stretches the spine, and works on strengthening the muscles in the back and stomach.

MINI TRIANGLE

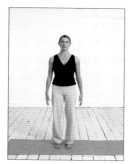 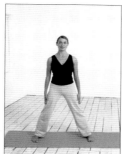 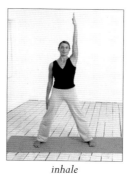 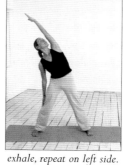

inhale

exhale, repeat on left side.

CHOPPING WOOD

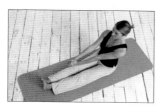 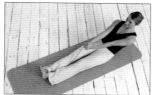 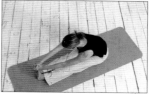

exhale

inhale

BIG STRETCH   ## THE BALL

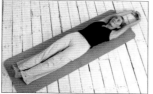 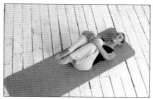

inhale

exhale

BRIDGE

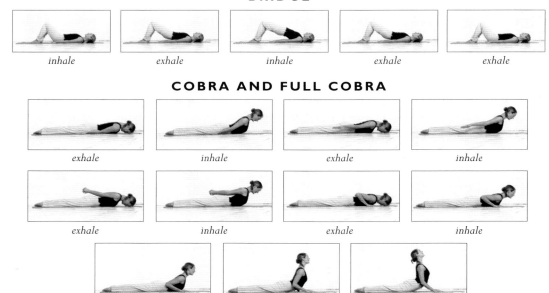

inhale   *exhale*   *inhale*   *exhale*   *exhale*

COBRA AND FULL COBRA

exhale   *inhale*   *exhale*   *inhale*

exhale   *inhale*   *exhale*   *inhale*

inhale   *inhale*   *inhale*

EXTENDED CAT AND MOVING FROM THE COBRA
TO THE CHILD'S POSE

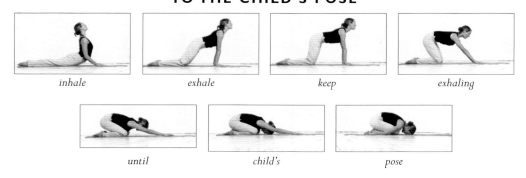

inhale   *exhale*   *keep*   *exhaling*

until   *child's*   *pose*

CHILD'S POSE

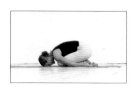

CALM

If ever you just want to calm down, yoga is perfect. The most important thing is to really use the breathing to slow down your thoughts and relax the body. There are not many postures within this plan, so you should concentrate on holding the postures for long periods. The Seated Forward Bend (see page 70) is a great posture for just giving up and letting go. A breathing technique is included here, but please use your common sense when doing it. If your nostrils are completely blocked then simply try deep breathing to clear your passages.

CHILD'S POSE

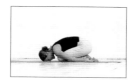

NECK RELEASE

 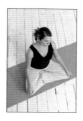 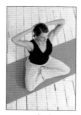 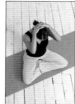

inhale   *exhale*

SHOULDER ROLLS

inhale   *inhale*   *exhale*

EXTENDED CAT AND MOVING FROM THE COBRA
TO THE CHILD'S POSE

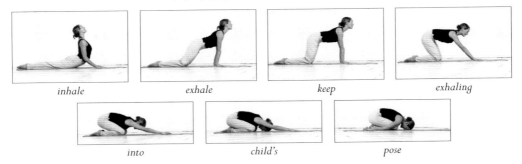

inhale   *exhale*   *keep*   *exhaling*

into   *child's*   *pose*

INVERTED V

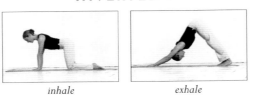

inhale   *exhale*

SEATED FORWARD BEND

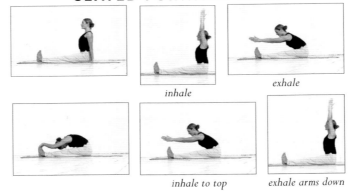

inhale   *exhale*

inhale to top   *exhale arms down*

BREATHING EXERCISES

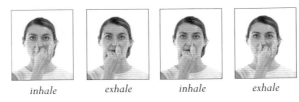

inhale   *exhale*   *inhale*   *exhale*

Some Help From Shiatsu

Each body has the innate and miraculous ability to heal itself. The body's vital force runs in specific energetic pathways called meridians in Chinese medicine and nadis in Yoga. These meridians are intimately linked to the healthy functioning of our internal organs. If energy flow becomes obstructed, the body's balance is disrupted and illness results. Shiatsu uses finger, elbow and knee pressure, gentle stretching and energetic body work to remove blockages and bring balance and harmony back to the body and mind and spirirt.

Press on each point for 10 rounds of breath unless directed otherwise.

HEADACHES IN THE EYES AND TEMPLES

Press fairly gently in the webbing of the foot, between the large and second toe metatarsals. Follow this by squeezing the inside of the big toe just below the nail. This may hurt a little but it releases the stagnant liver energy causing the headache.

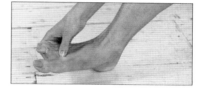

SINUS HEADACHES AND GENERAL WELL-BEING

This is a great one to do daily. It takes the energy out of the head and down to the feet, grounding you, which is obviously great for a headache. I also use this one when I have a lot of chatter in my head – it really works. It also drains the lymphatic system.

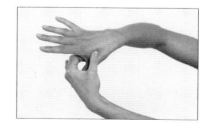

Press fairly hard into the webbing of the hand, between thumb and first finger. It will probably feel a little uncomfortable.

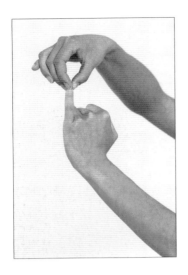

ENERGY, HEALTH

Pressing daily on these points in each finger and toe will help keep the energy moving freely through your body, maintaining good health.

Taking your first finger and thumb, squeeze either side of your nail at the bottom for a few seconds, release and move on to the next. Don't be really gentle, you are trying to release your energy.

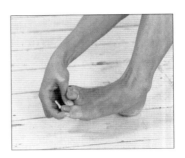

STOMACH BLOATING AND NUTRITIONAL PROBLEMS

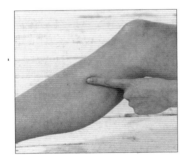

This is a real help when you still feel uncomfortable some time after eating.

Go down the inside of the leg, next to the shinbone. Follow the picture so you don't go too far down – there is an obvious natural hollow and this is the point. Press and hold.

AEROPLANE PRESSURE WITH THE EARS

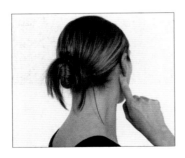

If you're on a plane and your ears don't unblock, this can help to release the pressure.

Take your first finger behind the earlobe – have a close look at the picture – and firmly press. It will probably be a little uncomfortable. Do this on both sides.

PERIOD CRAMPS

The first three pictures are the preparations to get you into the correct position to help alleviate cramps. Pressure here gets the blood flowing in this area; when it becomes stagnant cramps occur.

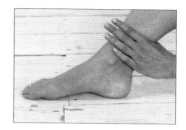

You might be better off getting someone to help you with this one, as it can be awkward to get the right positions. Please do it on both legs and hold it for longer than the rest — perhaps even for 5–10 minutes. You are looking for a balanced pulse between the two points eventually, using very gentle pressure. It's best to do this before extreme cramping but it will still work if you have gone beyond that point.

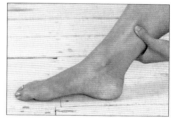

Take four fingers up from the top of your anklebone. You'll find the right point where the fourth finger is, just inside the shinbone.

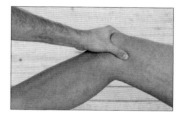

Take your other hand with your fingers together and stretch out your thumb. Following the picture, your hand will find a natural place on top of the kneecap where it should feel very comfortable. It took me a few attempts to get this right, so keep practising. It should fit like a glove. Notice where the thumb is on this area as this is the correct point.

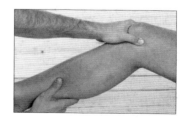

Putting it all together is the actual point. Remember to do both legs!

Now Where?

Okay, you have done all the postures and the breathing techniques and you want more. Slow down. Yoga is all about relaxation and comfort, and there is never any hurry. Do you really feel completely relaxed and comfortable in each posture? Are you able to hold the position and keep your mind on the breathing at the same time? If so, great! But if not, and if you are not yet stretching into the full posture (as I have tried to demonstrate in the pictures) then take your time. I have attempted to give you the essential tools for a firm foundation for any future practice of yoga, take your time and enjoy the full benefits of what is shown here before you try looking for more.

If you are ready to move on then there are two ways to go about it.

The first is to continue learning at home. This takes a lot of discipline and hard work, but if you have reached this point then hopefully you will have built up a good routine by now, so that shouldn't be a problem. The reason it is so hard is that you don't have a teacher to correct you, and many of the more advanced postures could actually be dangerous if done incorrectly. Find a good teaching book or video (there are too many for me to list here) and really focus on making sure you understand each posture before actually trying it. In advanced postures most of the pressure is normally on the spine, be really careful and aware of this.

The second way is the way I would recommend which involves finding a class and learning the more advanced postures from a qualified teacher. There are plenty of yoga classes around and often the hardest thing is deciding which one to choose.

One good piece of advice is that if you do find a teacher, then try to do an actual course. Most courses run from 8 to 12 weeks and are a great way to learn new postures, meet new people and really get to know how the teacher works. From that point your teacher would probably be the best person to advise you on further practice.

Below is a pretty basic guide to how to choose a class.

GYM OR YOGA CENTRE?

Classes are everywhere now and location is not always a guarantee that you will find a good teacher. Look around and just see if you find something that appeals to you, whether for convenience or just because it sounds good, but be prepared to look elsewhere if you don't feel comfortable after a class or two. This is all about you so find the one that feels right. If you know someone who does yoga then have a chat with them, they may know a good teacher you can try.

WHAT TYPE OF YOGA?

This is where it can get tricky. Yoga classes are called by all kinds of names and I have tried to give a quick guide to what you can expect in some of the more usual styles.

IYENGAR YOGA

Created by Mr Iyengar, this type of yoga is very precise and technically correct, with focus on building power through proper alignment of the body. There is not really one set sequence that is taught, and you may do some postures with a variety of ropes, blocks and chairs. A good Iyengar teacher can make you feel a foot taller!!

SIVANANDA YOGA

Named after Swami Sivananda, movement, flow and relaxation are the foundations of Sivananda Yoga. Classes begin with the Sun Salutation, and then a set sequence of twelve postures are taught. The postures vary in difficulty and the entire sequence is thought to stretch every major muscle group in every direction. Relaxation is central, especially between postures. Sivananda classes always make me feel completely relaxed.

ASHTANGA YOGA

Mr Pattabi Jois invented Ashtanga Yoga, and it is a rigorous and powerful sequence that uses deep breathing through the throat to increase the 'fire' in the body. Postures are held for long periods and the Sun Salutation is performed with a powerful jump back. Throughout the postures the deep breathing builds up heat all over, generating sweat and a great burn for the body.

OTHER TYPES OF YOGA

Well, there are hundreds but the three explained above are probably the most widely taught in the West. Remember, if it is Hatha Yoga it is physical yoga so if you see a class you want to attend and the style is alien to you, just ask them whether it is a type of Hatha Yoga. If it is, then at least you know you will be doing postures that you will probably recognize, although they may be taught differently.

Good luck and, remember, enjoy . . .

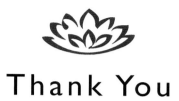

Thank You

To my teachers Niriyani and Barbara for setting me on this extraordinary path with such compassion and love. I smile each day. Thank you.

To my ever inspiring students.

This is a chance to put down some words to my Rippy. Without her continuing support through my life since I was knee high, I wouldn't be here writing this. We've come a long way on this amazing journey, haven't we? I treasure you and although your arms are always wrapped around me, Mum, mine will always be wrapped around you. In my heart. X

Dad, I know you look on silently proud. Thank you, thank you for always encouraging me and being there, believing in me and supporting me. Now's the time to look after you!

My big brother Markie – since lending me your sparkling blue eyes a whole new world has opened up to me. I feel you watching over me, thank you for guiding me. I just wish that you were here – I know that I'm not the only one. One day though, eh boy?

Scobie for being so amazing and patient with your little sis through the years and introducing me to my lovely sister-in-law Angelica and my gorgeous niece and nephew, Jessica and Luke.

My two Nans who I miss, but I know that you're watching. Kisses xxxxx.

To all my family and relatives, godparents as well, thank you for your continuing love.

LJ that Boy, Love you!

And all my dear friends: Rachy button moon, I love ya more than . . . Baby Poppy, you're a lucky girl to have picked a special mummy like that, Missy my Smealie for all the madness that we have experienced already in such a short life, thinking of you always makes my heart smile. J Boa, Sheeps and baby V, Scobie louy doo, Louy and by the time this book is published small person too! Jump and the boys, one of them being my beautiful godson. Tanya and Jake and all my fellow yogis from Sunra 99. JB for always being there xxx I treasure that! To my friend, Sarah — when I think of you I'm smiling and waving at you with a sparkle in my eyes. To Paul, Mr Collins — without you this book wouldn't have been possible, thank you for being my rock on this one. Ruby, Alice and mad Bentley and to the lovely Sally because if it hadn't been for your karma, I certainly wouldn't be doing this. To the lovely Geri for changing my journey, big kiss back. Ingrid for approaching me on this project — we've had good fun haven't we, Mr Prebble and Mr Benedict, glad you're here!!! Dr Alla and Galina for opening up a whole new world to me. Brendan for showing me a rainbow, Anamai, Manuel and Ines for your constant support and anyone I have missed.

Namaste beautiful people in my life.

I'm a lucky girl.

Peace

Om